INNOVATIONS IN PAEE

A Nursi

Other books edited by Edward Alan Glasper

Child Care – Some Nursing Perspectives (1991)

Advances in Child Health Nursing (1993) (with Ann Tucker)

Whaley & Wong's Children's Nursing (1995) (with Stephen Campbell)

INNOVATIONS IN PAEDIATRIC AMBULATORY CARE

A Nursing Perspective

Edited by

Edward Alan Glasper and Susan Lowson

MACMILLAN

First published 1998 by
MACMILLAN PRESS LTD
Houndmills, Basingstoke, Hampshire RG21 6XS
and London
Companies and representatives throughout the world

ISBN 0–333–68478–8 paperback

A catalogue record for this book is available from the British Library.

This book is printed on paper suitable for recycling and made from
fully managed and sustained forest sources.

10 9 8 7 6 5 4 3 2 1
07 06 05 04 03 02 01 00 99 98

Editing and origination by
Aardvark Editorial, Mendham, Suffolk

Printed in Malaysia

CONTENTS

NOTES ON CONTRIBUTORS

Maureen Ballentine is an experienced Hospital Play Specialist and is presently working as a Play Coordinator at Southampton University Hospitals NHS Trust.

Rachel E Bia is a Lecturer/Practitioner at the Children's Trust in Tadworth, Surrey.

Michael A Cooper is a Lecturer/Practitioner in Child and Adolescent Mental Health Nursing based at the University of Southampton's School of Nursing and Midwifery.

Ruth Davis fulfils the dual role of Diabetes Care Coordinator and Honorary Lecturer in Nursing at the University Hospital of Wales, Cardiff.

Margaret Evans is a former Lecturer in Paediatric Oncology Nursing and Nurse Consultant at the University of Southampton's School of Nursing and Midwifery.

Yvonne Fulton is a Teaching Fellow in Child Health Nursing at the University of Southampton's School of Nursing and Midwifery.

Edward Alan Glasper is Professor of Nursing and Director of Child Health Studies at the University of Southampton's School of Nursing and Midwifery.

Diane Gow is a Teaching Fellow in Child Health Nursing at the University of Southampton's School of Nursing and Midwifery.

Louise Hooker is the Wessex Cancer Trust Lecturer in Paediatric Oncology Nursing at the University of Southampton's School of Nursing and Midwifery.

Lorraine Ireland is a Lecturer in Child Health Nursing at the University of Southampton's School of Nursing and Midwifery.

Susan Jones is a Ward Manager at Bristol Royal Hospital for Sick Children and is also Chairperson of the RCN Society of Paediatric Nursing.

Paulajean Kelly was a former Clinical Nurse Specialist in Research within Tower Hamlets Paediatric Home Care Team, London. Her current post is as a Lecturer in Children's Nursing at City University.

Lesley Lowes is a Paediatric Diabetes Specialist Nurse at the Department of Child Health, University Hospital of Wales, Cardiff.

Susan Lowson is Quality Development Manager at the Southampton University Hospitals NHS Trust and former Senior Clinical Nurse to the Child Health Directorate.

Rachel McWilliams is a Family Information Nurse in the Children's Outpatient Department at the Southampton University Hospitals NHS Trust.

Sarah Palmer is a Paediatric Oncology Nurse at the Piam Brown Unit, within the Child Health Directorate of the Southampton University Hospitals NHS Trust.

Deborah Perriment is a former Child Protection Nurse Specialist at Southampton University Hospitals NHS Trust.

Linda Phillips is Manager of the Children's Outpatient Department within the Southampton University Hospitals NHS Trust.

Catherine Powell is a Child Protection Nurse Specialist within the Southampton University Hospitals NHS Trust and a lecturer in Child Health Nursing at the University of Southampton's School of Nursing and Midwifery.

Jim Richardson is Lecturer in Child Health Nursing at the University of Wales College of Medicine, Cardiff.

Helen Rushforth is a Lecturer in Child Health Nursing at the University of Southampton's School of Nursing and Midwifery.

Jeanne Smith is a Research Nurse in the Department of Social Medicine, University of Bristol.

Sharon Stower is the Senior Nurse Manager of Children's Services at the Queen's Medical Centre, Nottingham.

Anne Thompson works at the Royal Victoria Infirmary, Newcastle, where she is a Paediatric Macmillan Nurse.

Valerie Wilkins was the Programme Co-ordinator of the Medical Information Centre at the Hospital for Sick Children, Toronto, Canada.

Stephen Wright was formerly a Visiting Professor of Nursing at the University of Southampton's School of Nursing and Midwifery, and he is the Director of The European Nursing Development Agency (TENDA).

FOREWORD

The care which we, as a society, offer to children is a fundamental reflection of the values which guide our lives. Hence within health-care the services which are developed for children should be at the forefront of development, drawing on wide-ranging knowledge which impinges not only on advances in medical technology but also on patterns of organisational care and personal, social and learning needs of children and their families. This text is to be welcomed since it blends these issues in such a way as to make them readily accessible to readers while pushing forward an understanding of new and innovative ways of providing care.

Neither ambulatory care nor the requirements to address children's needs within the context of their families is new. What may be seen as fresh is the progress which has been made on many fronts, which opens up a range of options which may not have been available in the past. Advances in telecommunications can overcome problems with access, blending the supportive educative skills of nursing with skilled diagnosis in nurse-led clinics can help to focus on problems which are meaningful to patients and their families, and providing access to information in a form which makes it accessible to those without a knowledge of healthcare fundamentally alters the relationship between care giver and recipient of care.

This leads me to one of the issues which I find most interesting, namely the shifting interrelations between both practitioners and patients and at an interdisciplinary level which are described in many of the chapters. First there is an underlying belief in the need to hold families together, to share care and information with them in order that a true partnership can be formed. Such a shift sounds simple but can easily become rhetoric. Yet it is fundamental to the manner in which relations are handled within the delivery of healthcare.

It is not only the relationships between health care workers and patients which are challenged. Further partnerships are demonstrated between nurses working in practice, education and research in such a way as to bring together these specialist areas of skill. Yet another crucial partnership can be seen in the relationships which are emerging between primary and secondary care. At a time when there is a growing emphasis on care in the community, it is essential that the patients receive care which calls on the best of both worlds, a service at home, offered by those who are skilled in community care but in partnership with the highly specialised skills of secondary and tertiary services.

The authors of this text do not suggest that they can offer all the answers to ambulatory care for children. Indeed it would be foolhardy to do so since developments are occurring so rapidly. They do, however, offer a diversity of approaches, drawing on a wealth of experience and knowledge which will, I have no doubt, act as a valuable stimulus for others.

Barbara Vaughan MSc DipN DANS RNT
Visiting Professor – University of Bournemouth
Programme Director – Nursing Developments King's Fund

PREFACE

Ambulatory care is one of the fastest growing branches of health care in Western societies. The transition from tertiary inpatient care (which began for children in 1852 with the opening of the Hospital for Sick Children, Great Ormond Street, London, and culminated in the building of large district general hospitals) to an essentially primary health care-led health service has created the conditions necessary for the development of ambulatory care services.

Ambulatory care is the vehicle that will bridge the euphemistic service provision gaps that prevent a seamless web of care being delivered to children and their families. This text seeks to focus on innovations within ambulatory care but is not exhaustive. Indeed, the various chapters fail to reflect adequately the full range of recent developments, which is perhaps a reflection of just how proactive children's nurses are within the field. There is no doubt that children's nurses have led the way in the design, implementation and evaluation of ambulatory care services for families.

The renewed energies of children's nurses within this arena are also indicative of the growth in specialisation linked to the clinical nurse specialist movement that has concentrated on the area of ambulatory care. The technical sophistication of tertiary medicine, coupled to the changing roles of junior doctors, has also been a causative factor in placing ambulatory care in the spotlight of change. Nurses have been quick to grasp and exploit these new opportunities to promote their expertise. Their commitment to partnership with families has influenced the strategic development of many ambulatory care services, and this book is a tribute to those many children's nurses who are working tirelessly to improve standards of care and who challenge practice.

This book is offered as a series of chapters exploring the unique contribution that children's nurses can make to developing ambulatory care within a diverse range of clinical settings. Chapter 1 examines the growth of ambulatory care from a historical perspective and details parameters of service delivery. Chapter 2 addresses the contentious issues of expanding roles within a paediatric A&E department, the area of ambulatory care most familiar to families given the evidence of childhood accidents. This chapter examines nurses' utilisation of skills more normally associated with doctors and documents the evolution of the A&E paediatric nurse practitioner. Chapters 3 and 4 examine the concept of information-giving as the key to family empowerment and debates the growing role of telecommunications as a vehicle to transmit information.

North American ambulatory care facilities now undergo accreditation by the Accreditation for Ambulatory Health Care Inc. Such accreditation emphasises the need for robust standards within the field of ambulatory care and highlights the importance of the discipline within the area of contemporary health care provision.

Chapter 5, which discusses the achievements of a King's Fund accredited nursing development unit situated within an outpatient department, is indicative of the profession's desire to develop services in the best interest of children and their families, and to ensure that 'families first' is the philosophy of care.

Chapter 6 concentrates on the medium of play and acknowledges the importance of therapeutic play in the overall delivery of ambulatory care and its function within the multidisciplinary team.

Chapters 7 and 8 investigate ambulatory care services for children with cancer and examine in detail the role played by paediatric Macmillan services.

Chapters 9 and 10 detail the growing phenomenon of nurse-led clinics and the development of clinical nurse specialism that has consistently linked itself to the growth in ambulatory care services.

Chapter 11, related to community nursing, is a timely reminder that less than 50 per cent of the UK is served by community paediatric nurses, despite the explicit recommendations of the NHS 'Children's Charter'. Paediatric community nursing services are destined to play a larger part in the development of ambulatory care services for children. It is, perhaps, a tribute to paediatric community nurses that advances in ambulatory care have, to a greater or lesser extent, been commensurate with their own success. A healthy primary health care service is essential if ambulatory care is not to become a euphemism for cost-cutting in cash-strapped health economies.

Chapter 12 concentrates on issues related to child protection. The victims of child abuse in its widest context are often first to be witnessed in an ambulatory care setting. The wide spectrum of abuse, which incorporates physical, sexual and emotional parameters, is likely to be a constant feature of some ambulatory care services, especially A&E departments. A sound knowledge of the protocols associated with child protection is an essential toolkit for the paediatric nurse working in an ambulatory care setting for it is here that the sharp end of deprivation is likely to be seen.

Chapter 13 considers the cultural sensitivities that paediatric nurses must process if they are successfully to harness the challenges of ambulatory care, and Chapter 14 relates the establishment of a community outreach programme for children with complex disabilities. It is often forgotten, or ignored, that children with the most complex of needs, that is, those with a learning difficulty and with or without profound physical disability, are at the sharp end of ambulatory care. The decline of longer-term institutional care long heralded in the professional press as the object of derision fails to recognise the sheer logistical problem for families attempting to care for their disabled children.

Chapter 15 examines the growth of paediatric day care long eulogised since the publication of the Court Report in 1976. The standard-bearer of ambulatory care, day care relies on many factors, principally a family able to cope.

Chapter 16 is very much a case study approach to a particular medical problem, which is growing in incidence among the childhood population. Diabetes is increasingly being managed in ambulatory care surroundings, thus avoiding inpatient stays.

Chapter 17 begins to address the management issues that have developed alongside the growth in ambulatory care. The 'hub and spoke' model described in this chapter should resolve some of the tensions and delineates the role of the differing sectors of the health care community.

Chapter 18 is the last chapter, but this is in no way intended to marginalise the subject matter, that is, mental health. This chapter, in using a case study approach, effectively concentrates the mind of the reader on the wide variety of psychological problems suffered by children and young people. Such children are managed in ambulatory care settings, and the result of the interactions, which are primarily nurse led, is a clear indicator of their success.

We hope you find the text a good introduction to the vast area of ambulatory care and that you find some of the descriptions of care both stimulating and inspiring. The cover illustration, *Journeying*, was chosen because of the nature of patients' progress through ambulatory care and the journey that inevitably occurs. *Journeying* is a textile, metal and glass artwork that was commissioned by the

Partnerships Art Programme on behalf of the Trust Chaplaincy Team for the Chapel at Southampton General Hospital. Faith and the experience of illness within life's journey were explored by the artist working with patients, staff and local community groups.

Local schoolchildren and inpatients from the children's wards were involved in the process. The birds show hope, energy, rebirth and celebration. The gold line that circles through the work indicates the lifeline and life's journey for the patient coping with transition and change. Areas where the lifeline crosses over another section indicate choice, decision-making and the opportunity for the patient to reflect – 'a time to think about the past and future questions'. The process of ambulatory care is constant for the patient, requiring flexibility and careful management. It is essential in all practice that the patients' and families' journeys are escorted by health care professionals constantly reviewing their practice and evaluating care.

E.A. GLASPER AND SUSAN LOWSON

1

AMBULATORY CARE – THE SCOPE OF PRACTICE

F A. Glasper and Susan Lowson

Ambulatory care is defined as 'health services provided on an outpatient basis to those who visit a hospital or clinic and depart after treatment on the same day' (Mosby, 1995). Once the backwater of hospital medicine, ambulatory care is now beginning to play a dominant role in the shop window of the health service in the UK and further afield.

Historical background

The father of ambulatory care for children, Dr George Armstrong, established the first recorded dispensary for the infant poor in London in 1769 (Alpert, 1995). The British Dispensary Movement during the eighteenth and first half of the nineteenth century reflected the lack of inpatient provision for sick children. This did not come into existence until 1852 with the opening of the Hospital for Sick Children, Great Ormond Street, London, the UK's first children's hospital. It is perhaps ironic that the father of paediatric ambulatory care was highly influential in delaying inpatient care for children, postulating that children and their parents should not be separated (Miles, 1986). Armstrong further believed that parents would not be able to look after their children in hospital because of economic pressures. In these respects, he was particularly prophetic, but not perhaps in the way he intended. It is the area of ambulatory care that is perhaps more economically debilitating for parents than is inpatient care.

The rapid move towards community care has catapulted ambulatory care into the spotlight of change. The transition from traditional outpatient care to modern ambulatory care has been challenging for many units who have found themselves ill prepared for change. Although professional children's nurses working in all areas of child care are now firmly committed to the concept of family-centred care and family advocacy, they have to reconcile the advantages of ambulatory care with the ability of parents to cope with the extra demands that this may entail.

Armstrong, with his famous quotation cited in many modern journal papers – 'To take a sick child away from its parents breaks its heart immediately' (Palmer, 1993) – was perhaps not fully appreciative of the appalling conditions in which children lived throughout this period of history. The slums of London so vividly described in the many novels of Charles Dickens, particularly in *Oliver Twist*, were a reality for the majority of children during the first half of the nineteenth century. Ambulatory care, which was the Dispensary Movement of that era, was insufficient to safeguard the health of children, and its failure to do so contributed to the opening of inpatient children's hospitals from 1852 onwards.

If poor ambulatory care provision was a contributory direct precursor of tertiary inpatient care for children in the nineteenth century, it must follow that excellence in tertiary care for children in the late twentieth century will be a precursor for the ascendency of ambulatory care in the twenty-first. Ambulatory care can, therefore, only flourish in a climate that has achieved, at least in terms expressive of good health, those objectives envisaged when the UK National Health Service (NHS) was created in 1947. Although health in late twentieth-century contemporary society is vastly different from that of the nineteenth century, it must not be assumed that the conditions that bred ill-health in its widest definition have disappeared. Far from it, for there remain elements of British post-industrial society that are as dangerous to child mental and physical health as were elements of nineteenth-century society, once described as the golden era of British capitalism.

It can be hypothesised that the transition of care from tertiary to ambulatory provision is still in its infancy, at least within the UK. Few would disagree that a robust primary health care service is essential if ambulatory care is to grow and prosper. Ambulatory care must not be seen in political terms as a cheap option for the care of children, although there are clearly fiscal benefits that accompany this development in care for Western governments.

The precursors to ambulatory care for children

Armstrong's views of inpatient care have been reiterated throughout the intervening years. The 1959 Welfare of Children in Hospital publication (Department of Health, 1959), a seminal document, proved to be a high watermark in the establishment of better care facilities for the families of sick children in hospital. The so-called Platt Report (after the Chairman, Sir Harry Platt) recommended that children should not be admitted to hospital unless absolutely necessary. Many of Platt's recommendations were based on the work of two pioneering child psychologists, John Bowlby and James Robertson, who articulated the pitfalls and negative psychological sequelae of an unaccompanied inpatient stay during childhood (Bowlby, 1951; Robertson, 1962). These laudable views must, however, be taken in context given that the potential dangers of non-hospital admission for children in the early days of antibiotic therapy would almost certainly have outweighed the potential psychological problems of an inpatient stay. Despite this caveat, generations of parents have expressed feelings of helplessness and inadequacy during their child's admission to hospital, when nurses have completely taken over their care.

This less than satisfactory state of affairs continued long after the publication of the Platt Report and did not improve substantially until after the founding of the National Association for the Welfare of Children in Hospital (NAWCH), now known as Action for Sick Children, in 1961. NAWCH accelerated the pace of change and became the champion of parents as consumers of health care; in many ways, it can be seen as echoing the voice of George Armstrong in campaigning for greater ambulatory care provision. While the Platt Report recommended that children should not be admitted unless absolutely necessary, there was little in the published text to promote ambulatory care. It is difficult to conceptualise how such a strategy might have been implemented in the absence of fundamental health policy change when there was little, if any, provision for the care of children in their own homes. The paediatric community nurse was still to be a future initiative.

Despite this, it is perhaps worthy of note that the current move towards day surgery, first reported in 1909 by Nicoll, was founded on the premise that the separation of a child from its mother might be harmful. This being so, it would almost certainly have been true that not separating a child from an environment that was a harbinger of disease would also have been harmful. In the early

3

years of the twentieth century, there were probably not many lower socioeconomic households in the UK where a child could have been successfully nursed at home following surgery. Although receiving little mention in the Platt Report (Department of Health, 1959) ambulatory care for children is implicit in the Court Report *Fit For the Future* (Department of Health, 1976).

Translating the rhetoric of government recommendations into action policy has taken decades, and the whole concept of day care provision for children has spread very slowly. The infrastructure to support a widespread embrace of ambulatory care philosophy is still being developed, and the seamless web of service envisaged in the Caring for Children in the Health Services' publication *Bridging the Gaps* (Thornes, 1993) is yet to be fully realised. Some of this is dependent upon a robust, efficient and effective paediatric community nursing service. Atwell and Gow (1985) have pioneered the recognition that caring for sick children can be managed at home and have thus paved the way for the development of paediatric community nursing services, at least in some UK community Trusts. Such services are far from universal, but at the very least form the foundation stones of ambulatory care services. The UK Children's Charter (NHS, 1996) published in 1996 expressly states that parents should have appropriate help and support from a community nursing team when their child requires care at home. Despite this clear commitment, there remain many areas of the UK that do not provide this service for the parents of sick children.

The increased use of day care services for children, coupled with earlier discharge from hospital, necessitates the development of a widely available paediatric community nursing service. The original driving force behind some such schemes was the need to provide care for children post-operatively following day surgery (Glasper *et al.*, 1989). Although this remains a high priority within many paediatric community teams, the repertoire of services has increased enormously, and much of the current trend in ambulatory care depends on their continued growth and development. This symbiotic relationship between a sophisticated primary health care sector and a decline in the need for tertiary inpatient care does not, however, always recognise that it is the parent who is the lynch pin in the provision of care for children, be they sick or well. Demographic changes in employment patterns are responsible for a strong female sector workforce with a corresponding decline in male sector employment. The continued availability of family structures necessary to underwrite continued growth in ambulatory care must therefore be questioned.

This notwithstanding, it must be recognised that, although many parents are able to deliver excellent nursing care to their sick children, there will be many situations and occasions when they may be incapable of doing so. In these situations, it is the partnership between the nurse and the family (Casey, 1995) that will underpin the continued success of family-centred care within the community. Rickard and Finn (1997) highlight the reality that parents are often in a position of identifying the onset of symptoms in a child as he or she becomes ill. This reality should prompt health care professionals to accelerate the move towards partnership in which the role of the practitioner is to empower the family to make its members more efficient in the management of childhood conditions. The continued growth in ambulatory care provision for children under the auspices of the current UK health service will require further investigation of the partnership paradigm if the term is not to become a euphemism for cost-cutting service re-engineering, a strategy that places the burden of care on families who may be as ill equipped to cope as were their Victorian ancestors. Although the coping strategies were necessarily different in this time period, what is different about twentieth-century family-centred care is the disenfranchisement of the family from normal life health events, such as major illnesses, birth, deaths and other such crises, that were so common in the homes of Victorian families.

Family-centred care

The re-education of families in the provision of care to family members has been described by St John and Rolls (1996). They link the growth in tertiary inpatient care with the decline in the ability of families to cope with members who are ill. The nursing profession may, however, have underestimated the power of the family to act as an important deliverer of care. Only in harnessing this latent care provision will ambulatory care achieve the growth rate to which it aspires. The explosion in surgical and medical day care facilities for children is perhaps the most visible avenue that ambulatory care has taken since the publication of the Court Report of 1976 (Department of Health, 1996). Thornes' important work on behalf of Caring for Children in the Health Services (Thornes, 1991) was inspired by the enthusiasm related to day care and the widespread belief that admitting children as day patients was an excellent way of providing good care. This was based on the prevailing philosophy of keeping children within their families, parents remaining the principal carers. Although Thornes' enquiry demonstrated that day care is an excellent strategy in dealing with many childhood problems, it nevertheless concluded that the process requires careful planning to avoid unnecessary stress on children and their families. It must be emphasised that ambulatory day care children do not only fall into a surgical category, but that day care also incorporates those children requiring medical interventions or investigations.

Perhaps the most important precursor of the development of ambulatory care for children in the closing years of the twentieth century is the Department of Health publication *Welfare of Children and Young People in Hospital* (Department of Health, 1991) and The House of Commons Health Committee reports (HMSO, 1997). The cardinal principle embodied within these documents is that children are admitted to hospital only if the care they require cannot be so well provided at home, in a day clinic or on a day basis in hospital. The far-reaching recommendations of this welfare document provide detailed guidelines for those involved with the care of children in A&E departments and day care units, among others. The publication of the welfare document coincided with the evolution of the purchaser/provider split within the UK health service, and it provided blueprints for the contracting of integrated patterns of child health care. Thus ambulatory care has begun to develop a higher profile.

The growth of ambulatory care

The Audit Commission report of 1993, entitled *Children First. A Study of Hospital Services*, has demonstrated that one child in four in the population attends an A&E department in any one year. Thus, for many children, their first contact with a hospital is through an A&E department. This makes A&E services the largest component of the ambulatory care sector of the health service. Despite these high attendance figures, A&E departments, in common with other areas of ambulatory care service, have not universally embraced the concept that children should have separate facilities. In an era when it is rare to find children being nursed with adults in inpatient settings, it is all too common to find A&E departments, outpatient departments and day care wards still following this pattern. This situation is lamentable, and the challenge of the Audit Commission report (1993) is for those who provide or intend to provide ambulatory care facilities for children to implement the principles of child- and family-centred care. This will require some reallocation of resources but more importantly a change in attitude of staff towards ambulatory care provision. The British Paediatric Association (now the College of Child Health) discussion document *Flexible Options for Paediatric Care – a Discussion Document* (1993) supports the move towards greater ambulatory paediatrics.

Perhaps the greatest precursor of the transition of ambulatory care from poor relation to flagship enterprise was the publication of the NHS Management Executive Value for Money Unit publication *Outpatient Departments – Changing the Skill Mix* (Kelly and Taylor, 1990), in which major changes to the way in which outpatient departments operate were suggested. The implied suggestions embodied within this report galvanised many units into action. Some units, such as the Child Health Directorate at Southampton, used the information in this publication to focus their audit activities and subsequently re-evaluated the role and future of paediatric nurses in an outpatient setting. Other paediatric units, such as Nottingham, began to lead the way in the development of innovative outpatient services for children (Stower, 1991), transforming the traditional environment associated with low-status nursing to one in which nursing began to demonstrate greater versatility and competence.

The stark choice facing children's outpatient department nurses, following the publication of the skill mix document, was to innovate or perish. Units such as Nottingham and Southampton continued to re-evaluate the contribution of paediatric nurses to the emerging ambulatory care discipline. Paediatric nurses remain keenly aware of their unique role in the care of children and their families and have responded positively to the rapid emergence of ambulatory care as a discrete discipline. Within the span of a few short years, the paediatric nursing profession has reacted to the ambulatory care challenge and has positively responded in a way that has addressed in a forthright manner those criticisms of its former mode of care delivery. The criticisms were undoubtedly justifiable – ambulatory care in one of its former guises as an outpatient service was the area of low status in nursing terms, the area in which to relocate those nurses who were deemed unsuitable for the higher-status inpatient care, those nurses who were musculoskeletally damaged: the 'bad backs' of the profession. It is perhaps fortunate that the professional aspirations of nursing have coincided with the growth in ambulatory care. Stower's description of the nurse-led clinics at Nottingham and the explicit Nottingham children's charter standards, which pre-date the publication of the NHS Children's Charter (NHS, 1996), are evidence of the willingness of paediatric nurses to adapt to changes in service provision for children and their families.

Clinical nurse specialism and ambulatory care

In addition, the evolution of the clinical nurse specialist has had an enormous influence on the development of paediatric ambulatory care nursing. 'Specialism/advanced practice' and 'nurse consultant' are terms that lack clarification but are often used interchangeably. Terms such as 'clinical nurse specialist' have gradually crept into the language of nursing over the past 10 years and have become part of the nomenclature associated with the profession. Although practice nurses in primary health care have led the way, it is the field of ambulatory care that has seen the most rapid development of clinical nurse specialism. In some countries, principally North America, ambulatory care clinical nurse specialists have to be Master's-degree prepared. This is helping to redress the balance of history, where it was the least qualified nurses, rather than the best, who worked in the area. Specialism in paediatric ambulatory care nursing has followed the growth of medicine as it has become increasingly mechanistic.

However, paediatric nurses have embraced specialism not because of medical expediency, especially in the light of the crisis caused by the reduction in junior doctors' hours of duties, but instead to promote the art and science of nursing. As Jacox and Norris (1977) have stated, 'Nursing is not second class medicine but first class health care.' In a similar vein, ambulatory nursing care is not second-class care but an area of excellence in practice. The emerging ambulatory care nurse specialists do not see their role as providing high-tech care at the expense of psychosocial care, and during this, the early years of their development, it will be important that such roles are firmly rooted in paediatric nursing rather than in medicine. The rapid introduction of ambulatory care nurse-led clinics makes such a stance vital, but there are still some who believe that the further development of the paediatric clinical nurse specialist will only fragment the patient and his family along medical model lines.

The seminal publication *Child Health Rights* (British Paediatric Association, 1995) has much within it for those seeking further to develop ambulatory care facilities for children and their families. In particular, the environment for health care is highlighted, and specific guidelines related to clinic times, protected areas for children, confidentiality and health promotion are detailed.

The environment for ambulatory care

The environment of ambulatory care areas such as A&E and outpatient departments has traditionally been neglected, and they are often dull, uninviting and even frightening places for children. Some areas that have not developed separate children's ambulatory care services often expose children to hostile sights and sounds. Some Canadian children's hospitals, such as the Children's Hospital of Eastern Ontario, have responded positively to the challenge of ambulatory care and have developed extremely sophisticated day attendance services. The creation of a non-threatening environment for children is evident in the infrastructure of the ambulatory care department. The design of this outpatient department was crystallised by Carlyle Designs Associates, a young company specialising in interior design for children's hospitals. Fronted by Anne Carlyle, the company has expertise in the design of public environments, concentrating on progressive environments for children. The firm's designs are comprehensive and multidisciplinary, including interior space planning, design, furniture and special product design and graphics, and exhibit and signage designing. Signage is particularly important in health care institutions, and bold imaginative strategies are necessary if families are to benefit positively from the hospital experience. It is a salutary fact that good design and use of colour costs no more than poor design and poor colour choice. Brown plastic chairs, battleship grey-painted walls and the absence of toys are not conducive to a positive visit to any institution.

It is widely believed that the physical environment of an ambulatory care area can have an important influence on child development, noise and crowding being reputed to have negative influences. The beneficial effects of an enriched environment are particularly important, given that children develop by interacting with the social and physical world in which they live. Children live in the here and now, and movement, sound, forms, colour, light, odour and touch are of great importance when designing a child-centred environment. Paediatric ambulatory care areas should be the hub of the child-centred wheel, where it is possible to provide opportunities for children to learn to move and to learn by moving. This will maximise motor capabilities within safe tolerable limits, instead of having the usual institutional aim of stopping children's movements by eliminating physical activities such as running and jumping.

Therapeutic play in ambulatory care areas

Although the use of play specialists within inpatient settings is widespread, the employment of play specialists within the arena of ambulatory care is less well developed. Hospitals such as the Hospital for Sick Children, Toronto, Canada, have extensive child life (play/education) departments, and there is full coverage within the ambulatory care areas. This cover extends to individual outpatient clinics, where the aim is to help children cope positively with the outpatient experience. The use of play specialists in all areas of ambulatory care, including A&E departments, should aim to create a situation that encourages children to participate in meaningful learning activities. Opportunities for constructive play can counteract the discomfort, boredom and frustration that are associated with long waits in ambulatory care areas.

The increasing use of ambulatory care settings for children's surgery has raised the profile of pre-admission programmes for children and their families. Such programmes aim to inoculate the children and their families against the stresses of the hospital experience. Ellerton (1994) evaluated a Canadian programme using a control and experiential group numbering, in total, 75 families. The results demonstrated that fewer children and parents in the programme group reported high anxiety levels while awaiting surgery. In a similar study, Glasper and Thompson (1993) reported that for some families, despite an invitation, attendance at the pre-admission programme was impossible for a variety of reasons. Attempts to improve attendance among the day case families, through the use of mailed personal invitations and information sheets, proved only partially successful. The ramifications of this for play specialists within ambulatory care are considerable, and a greater imaginative use of preparatory programmes on the day of the initial outpatient visit is required.

Paediatric ambulatory care as a developing area of nursing

Some ambulatory care units, such as those within the Southampton University Hospitals Trust Child Health Directorate, have demonstrated a proactive attitude towards the barrage of changes impacting on them. The staff at Southampton, rather than adopting a passive reactive attitude, applied to the London-based King's Fund for a grant to create a nursing development unit. The grant bid was shortlisted and was eventually successful in allowing the Southampton paediatric ambulatory care unit to become the UK's first paediatric outpatient nursing development unit (NDU). The status of 'nursing development unit' has facilitated an acceleration of change that would probably have taken much longer without the pump-priming benefit of the NDU award. Lowson (1995) has described the development of the paediatric NDU and discusses the ambulatory care staff's commitment to change and innovation with the aim of promoting family advocacy. The benefits of NDU status have allowed the unit to become the shop window for innovations throughout the Southampton Child Health Directorate (Campbell *et al.*, 1992).

Stower (1993) highlights, in discussing the benefits of quality measurement, the reflective element of innovations in ambulatory care provision for children. The modern health services of the Western world are now firmly committed to the concept of evidence-based care. Therefore, any children's nurses embarking on the path of change must build into their studies the appropriate evaluative techniques necessary to generate the data that will provide the evidence of its efficacy. Without such evidence, it is unlikely that innovative schemes will secure long-term funding.

The scope of ambulatory care provision for children and their families

This textbook is intended to explore some of the key developments in ambulatory care provision for children and their families in the UK and elsewhere. It is not an exhaustive text, and new developments are constantly evolving. The challenge of ambulatory care is only just beginning, and, as with many new disciplines, the academic base remains fluid and relatively unwritten. It is hoped that the following chapters will help the reader to explore the differing and emerging facets of this developing field of paediatric nursing, which is becoming greater than the sum of its parts.

It is perhaps fitting that this chapter, which began with Dr George Armstrong and the past, should return to the past and examine the role of the domiciliary nurse of the same period. Anne Marie Rafferty (Rafferty, 1995) gives a fascinating insight into why the hospital became the dominant focus for nursing care in the mid-nineteenth century, using the fictional character Nurse Sarah Gamp, created by Charles Dickens in his 1844 novel *Martin Chuzzlewitt* to illustrate the character denigration of the nineteenth-century domiciliary nurse. Rafferty argues that the medically orchestrated character assignation of the independent ambulatory care nurses of the period caused a loss of nursing autonomy, which nurses have been trying to reacquire ever since. Perhaps this new age of ambulatory care will help nurses to regain their lost autonomy and recover the independence of their nursing ancestors in the provision of care for the families of sick children.

References

Alpert, J.M. (1995) Paediatric history. The ambulatory pediatric association. *Pediatrics*, **95**(3): 422–6.

Atwell, J.D. and Gow, M.A. (1985) Paediatric trained district nurses in the community; expensive luxury or economic necessity. *British Medical Journal*, **291**: 227–9.

Audit Commission (1993) *Children First. A Study of Hospital Services.* (London: HMSO).

Bowlby, J. (1951) *Maternal Care and Mental Health.* World Health Organisation Monograph Series No. 2. (Geneva: WHO).

British Paediatric Association (1995) *Child Health Rights. Implementing the UN Convention on the Rights of the Child within the Health Service – A Practitioners Guide.* (London: BACCH).

British Paediatric Association, Health Services Committee (1993) *Flexible Options for Paediatric Care – A Discussion Document.* (London: BPA).

Campbell, S., Lowson, S. and Glasper, A. (1992) Families first: the Southampton NDU. *Paediatric Nursing*, **4**(8): 6–9.

Casey, A. (1995) Partnership nursing: influences on involvement of informal carers. *Journal of Advanced Nursing*, **22**: 1058–62.

Department of Health (1959) *Welfare of Children in Hospital* (Platt Report). (London: HMSO).

Department of Health (1976) *Fit for the Future* (Court Report). (London: HMSO).

Department of Health (1991) *Welfare of Children and Young People in Hospital.* (London: HMSO).

Ellerton, M.I.. (1994) Preparing children and families psychologically for day surgery: an evaluation. *Journal of Advanced Nursing*, **19**: 1057–62.

Glasper, E.A. and Thompson, M. (1993) Preparing children for hospital, in Glasper, E.A. and Tucker, A. (eds) *Advances in Child Health Nursing*. (London: Scutari Press).

Glasper, A., Gow, M. and Yerrell, P. (1989) A family friend. *Nursing Times*, **85**(4): 63–5.

Health Committee (1997) *The Specific Health Needs of Children and Young People*, Vol. I. (London: HMSO).

Jacox, A.K. and Norris, C.M. (1977) *Organising for Independent Nursing Practice*. (New York: Appleton & Cushing Crofts).

Kelly, T.A. and Taylor, B.P. (1990) *Outpatient Departments – Changing the Skill Mix*. (London: NHSME, UFM Unit Study Team).

Lowson, S. (1995) The growth of an NDU in a paediatric outpatient department. *British Journal of Nursing*, **4**(1): 36–8.

Miles, I. (1986) The emergence of sick children's nursing before the turn of the century. Part I. *Nurse Education Today*, **7**(2): 82–7.

Mosby (1995) *Mosby's Pocket Dictionary of Nursing Medicine and Professions Allied to Medicine* (London: Mosby).

NHS (1996) *The Patient's Charter Services for Children and Young People*. (London: HMSO).

Nicoll, J.H. (1909) The surgery of infancy. *British Medical Journal*, **11**: 753.

Palmer, S.J. (1993) Care of sick children by parents: a meaningful role. *Journal of Advanced Nursing*, **18**: 185–91.

Rafferty, A.M. (1995) The anomaly of autonomy: space and status in early nursing reform. *International History of Nursing Journal*, **1**(1): 43–5.

Rickard, S. and Finn, A. (1997) Parental knowledge of paediatric infectious diseases. *Ambulatory Child Health*, 13–19.

Robertson, J. (1962) *Hospitals and Children, A Parent's Eye View*. (London: Victor Gollancz).

St John, W. and Rolls, C. (1996) Teaching family nursing: strategies and experiences. *Journal of Advanced Nursing*, **23**: 91–6.

Stower, S. (1991) A quality service for children in the outpatient setting. *International Journal of Health Care Quality Assurance*, **4**(6): 4–9.

Stower, S. (1993) Innovative practice in the outpatient setting, in Glasper, E.A. and Tucker, A. (eds) *Advances in Child Health Nursing*, **4**: 41–53.

Thornes, R. (1991) *Just for the Day. Caring for Children in the Health Services*. (London: NAWCH).

Thornes, R. (1993) *Bridging the Gaps. Caring for Children in the Health Services*. (London: Action for Sick Children).

2

EXPANDING ROLES AND PRACTICE WITHIN PAEDIATRIC A&E DEPARTMENTS – THE CHILDREN'S NURSE PRACTITIONER

Susan J. Jones and Jeanne M. Smith

Every year, about a quarter of the child population of the UK will attend an A&E department. Some of these children will have relatively minor illnesses or injuries, but, regardless of the nature or severity of their presenting complaint, it is vital that they have access to specialist facilities and appropriately trained staff. Many hospitals have responded to patient need by reviewing service provision and extending the scope of nursing practice in order to meet the needs of all client groups, but in paediatric emergency care, the evolution of the children's nurse practitioner role has the potential to improve effective care for children and their families in the A&E department. Before looking more closely at this role and the challenges that such service developments present, it is worth looking at the background to children's attendances at A&E departments and the current state of emergency paediatric provision.

Children and A&E

The children and families who attend A&E departments (Figure 2.1) come with a wide variety of illnesses and injuries, and their care needs may be acute or life threatening, or may fall into those categories that could be managed by the primary health care team. However, regardless of the nature or severity of their illness or injury, it is well established that the health care needs of children and their families differ greatly from those of adults, and that children up to the age of 16 need a service provision different from that of adults within inpatient areas (Department of Health, 1991; Audit Commission, 1993).

- 3 million children in England and Wales attend A&E annually
- Children under 16 years represent 25–30 per cent of all cases seen
- Specialist/inner city units may have a 45 per cent paediatric caseload

Figure 2.1 Children's attendances at A&E departments (British Paediatric Association, 1988; Royal College of Nursing, 1995a, and b)

However, in many A&E departments, these recommendations (Figure 2.2) have yet to be implemented, although Partridge's (1997) study suggests that many departments may be in the process of reviewing their paediatric A&E facilities in the light of the Children's Charter. It is still a matter of disappointment that, although the latest Audit Commission report, *By Accident or Design* (Audit Commission, 1996), covers children's services, it fails to include guidelines for improvements in children's emergency care in its recommendations.

- Effective and prompt treatment with clear policies and protocols
- Child- and family-centred care with parental access at all times
- Staff specially qualified and skilled in the care of children
- Separate facilities that are appropriately equipped
- Appropriate admission and effective communication with other staff and agencies on discharge

Figure 2.2 Appropriate provision for children in A&E departments – key recommendations from *Children First. A Study of Hospital Services* (Audit Commission, 1993)

The importance of appropriate facilities cannot be overemphasised, but the need for children's nurses who possess the appropriate skills and expertise in this field of nursing is of paramount significance. The Department of Health (1991) recommendation of every A&E department having at least one children's nurse on duty 24 hours a day is still far from being implemented, and in the units surveyed by the

Audit Commission (1996), none of the departments was able to meet this standard. Although there are eight specialist paediatric A&E units, the vast majority of children and young people will attend a general accident unit and are therefore likely to be nursed by registered general nurses who have been trained in the care of the adult.

A key issue in responding to the needs of children in the A&E department must surely be in the development of education and training courses designed specifically to address the care of children in the A&E department, as few such courses currently exist. It has been common practice to second children's nurses to the ENB 199 course, which has comparatively little paediatric content and, while it may cover some general principles, cannot address the sometimes complex needs of the child and family requiring emergency care, let alone provide adequate knowledge of the specific physiological, emotional, psychological and developmental needs of each age group.

When children's nurses are appointed to A&E departments, they are often required to be as involved in the care of the adult client as in that of the child and are frequently appointed to junior positions where the inability to improve the service and develop an awareness of children's needs results in a 'token' acknowledgement of the guidelines and recommendations for best practice. This also raises issues of recruiting and retaining children's nurses to general A&E departments, where their knowledge, expertise and skills may be undervalued by their peers and by management (Bentley, 1995) and where they may be unwilling to accept the lower grade typically offered while they gain experience in the care of the adult as well as the child (Audit Commission, 1996).

The problems of inadequately educated or skilled staff to undertake the care of the child and the family in the A&E department is reflected in an ethnographic study by Dingwall and Murray (1983). They observed how A&E staff labelled patients and made decisions concerning who complied to the notion of the ideal patient and who broke the rules. Good patients were those who displayed interesting symptoms or were in need of highly technical care; those who fell into the category of 'rubbish' or 'boring' patients were those who were judged to be inappropriate attendees, such as the patient who sprained an ankle a week ago but chose that evening to attend, or the drunk at the end of the queue. Children seemed to fall automatically into the category of rule-breakers, but, unlike that of their adult equivalents, their care was prioritised. It is interesting to note that this was in response to a perceived need to discharge them as quickly as possible rather than being an attempt to respond promptly to the child's needs in a potentially hostile and threatening environment. Prioritising care in this way has been used as safety valve in the past, and the practice will no doubt continue in the future

Assessing children in A&E

Assessing and treating children in the A&E department is challenging for even the most experienced nurse, and staff need to have developed advanced and quick assessment skills (Figure 2.3) to facilitate the effective triage of paediatric patients and to avoid needing the safety valve. The triaging of children should be based on an immediate assessment by an appropriately trained and experienced nurse in order to detect potentially life-threatening conditions and determine priorities of care. Nurses who are not experienced in the care of children may find them hard to assess in A&E departments for many reasons: their symptoms may be more vague, and outwardly 'normal' vital signs may mask a deteriorating condition because of the child's apparent ability to maintain a homeostatic state of compensation for longer periods than the adult (Hazinski, 1992). Communication may be hampered by the child's age or developmental stage, and the subsequent response to illness or injury may be further influenced by previous experiences of health care. Successful and appropriate triage of children in the A&E department is only a part of the role of the children's trained nurse, and the skills and knowledge gained in this practice area can form the basis for the development of new roles that take nursing in new and exciting directions.

● A knowledge of the anatomical and developmental differences between children and adults
● Recognition of the critically ill or injured child – based on these principles
● The knowledge and skills to recognise those conditions which may lead to respiratory or cardiac arrest, and appropriate interventions
● The ability to communicate sensitively and effectively with parents and carers as well as children at a time when the whole family may be under stress
● An understanding of the unofficial rules of triage

Figure 2.3 The main requirements for successful paediatric triage (Thomas, 1992)

The emergency nurse practitioner – expanding the nursing role

The development of the first nurse practitioner programme in 1965 by Loretta Ford and Henry Silver was based on a 'nursing model focused on the promotion of health in daily living, growth and development for children in families, as well as the prevention of disease and disability' (Silver *et al.*, 1968). It can be traced to the problems identified in the USA in the 1960s, when social, educational and demographic factors resulted in inadequate primary health care treatment for children. The nurse practitioner role is now both firmly established and widely accepted, as is the ambulatory model of care, but the forces that initiated those radical changes in nursing practice in America in the 1960s are still as relevant in the UK in the 1990s.

The role of the emergency nurse practitioner (ENP) in the UK is one that has developed in response to several factors:

- the reduction in junior doctors' working hours
- difficulty in recruiting suitably qualified medical staff to A&E
- a national profile of an increasing number of emergency referrals
- increasing levels of patient dissatisfaction
- difficulties in accessing primary health care services.

These factors, in combination with the fact that not all patients who attend A&E need, or even expect, to see a medical practitioner, have resulted in the expansion of advanced nursing roles such as that of the ENP.

As in the USA, nurse practitioner roles have developed where need is greatest, resources scarce or the population particularly vulnerable, working at what Jordan (1993) calls the 'social frontier'. All of these categories can be found in the A&E department, and the authors propose that children are certainly a vulnerable population. Jordan (1993), having reviewed the US and the UK literature, concludes that nurse practitioners are able to:

- fill care 'gaps'
- provide lower-cost primary care in primary and ambulatory settings
- provide good quality care
- give consultations that are highly valued by the patient.

One of the main features of the ENP's role has been to assess and treat to conclusion certain categories of patient under locally agreed protocols without reference to a doctor. The Royal College of Nursing (RCN, 1993, p. 1) has defined an ENP as:

An A&E nurse with a sound nursing practice base in all aspects of nursing, and with formal post basic education in holistic assessment, in physical diagnosis, in prescription of treatment and in the promotion of health.

In the UK, ENPs have operated informally for many years in many accident departments. Formally developed and accepted roles that were research based developed in the late 1980s, Oldchurch Hospital in Romford claiming to have established the first UK ENP service in 1986 (Morris et al., 1989). Research by James and Pyrogos (1989) added further weight to the argument for this new role, and the result of their 'paper exercise' revealed that experienced A&E sisters who assessed patients on the same basis as the senior house officer recommended correct treatment in 298 cases with only a very small number of patients (12) being 'mismanaged'. The clinical decisions made by ENPs have been shown to be safe and effective (Cooper and Robb, 1996), and patients report high levels of satisfaction with the more relaxed style of consultation offered by nurse practitioners (South West Thames Regional NHS Executive, 1994).

Specialist A&Es such as ophthalmology departments and dedicated paediatric A&E units were considered to have the greatest scope for the development and expansion of the role of nurse practitioner, and this is probably attributable to the high levels of expertise developed by nurses working in these specialist fields. However, paediatric A&Es have been slow to develop these roles. An action research study by Jones (1996) examined the feasibility of experienced registered sick children's nurses becoming children's ENPs. Jones found a paucity of relevant literature and commented that a perceived lack of suitably qualified and experienced nurses who were able to operate at advanced levels of practice and decision-making had undoubtedly influenced the lack of innovative roles in emergency paediatrics. Known examples of such roles have been described in Bristol, Lewisham and Nottingham, with recent developments in Glasgow and Manchester. The Nottingham study was able to demonstrate that 5 per cent of children attending A&E were treated to conclusion by children's ENPs (Kobran and Pearce,

1991). These figures are impressive, because, as many studies have demonstrated, when new roles begin, there is initial caution and, as confidence grows, the scope for the role expands. Southend, a major A&E department, was able to demonstrate that its ENPs treated up to 10 per cent of all the caseload to conclusion, resulting in a 50 per cent reduction in the waiting time for other patients to see the doctor (Burgess, 1992). There can be little doubt that here was a role that was ripe for expansion and one which would admirably complement medical care.

The feasibility study by Jones (1996) in Bristol addressed the question of whether experienced children's nurses would be able to perform this role after suitable training, as anecdotal evidence had led her to believe that nurses were already undertaking some aspects of this role, but without education and validation by peers and medical colleagues. The role was felt to encompass the essential aspects of nursing described by the RCN in 1989 (Figure 2.4).

- Offering direct access to nursing care for those wanting such services, and ensuring that this form of care was directly available
- Nurses providing such a service having deeper and more sophisticated assessment skills, which would be enhanced by programmes of education and training, thus enabling them to provide direct care in illness and injury, and giving them the ability to promote and maintain health and well-being
- An autonomous nursing service that encompasses the responsibility for managing the whole health care episode for the patient, from acceptance to discharge, and the ability to refer to other agents

---

Figure 2.4 Key characteristics of autonomous nursing practice (Royal College of Nursing, 1989)

Training and education for new nursing roles

In the case of the child and family attending the A&E department for a relatively minor illness or injury, the service that a children's ENP could provide would incorporate all those aims outlined by the RCN and, at the same time, allow nurses to expand and develop their role while enhancing care and service delivery. However, one of the first problems identified in the setting up of such a scheme is the lack of training and education courses designed to fit the needs of the nurse practitioner working in acute and specialist settings. The United Kingdom Central Council for Midwives, Nurses and Health Visitors (UKCC), in its document *The Scope of Professional Practice* (1992), stressed the need for expanded and new nursing roles to be underpinned by sound educational frameworks in order to ensure safe practice, as well as practitioners accepting the accountability for any actions they take in the context of their enhanced practice domain.

While under the UKCC's guidance, it would appear that such roles as that of the paediatric nurse practitioner might be undertaken under the umbrella of extending the scope of practice, dissent has arisen within the profession over who should be accorded the title of nurse practitioner, and increasing concern has been expressed that such roles may be those of a second-rate doctor rather than a first-class nurse. The RCN cited the need for specific educational preparation for such roles in its definition of a nurse practitioner:

> The nurse practitioner requires an advanced comprehensive programme of education and training in theory and practice, which incorporates experience of dealing with clients under the guidance and mentorship of preceptors, and assessment of competence in key areas of the nurse practitioner role. (RCN IANE, 1989)

While those aspiring to undertake such advanced practice roles as that of the nurse practitioner may well have amassed a great deal of experience and clinical knowledge, most nurse education programmes do not contain the subject areas that may be needed in the nurse practitioner domain. It has been suggested that these may include not only the biological sciences, but also the elements of pharmacology and pathophysiology, and the knowledge and skills to undertake the physical examination and assessment of clients (Stilwell, 1988). However, when the nurse practitioner role is developed in a speciality area within acute services, and has, perforce, a narrow focus of service, the chances of accessing and validating suitable programmes of education and training are extremely limited. Thus the majority of the nurse practitioner schemes in the acute setting do not fit the RCN model and have needed to develop and deliver in-house programmes.

The development of the Bristol project

The authors were appointed to research and initiate this project, and, based on a review of the current research and literature, as well as anecdotal evidence from professional colleagues in the field, devised an outline scheme to prepare and supervise children's ENPs in a specialist paediatric setting that combined acute, primary and ambulatory care. This planning stage was greatly enhanced by the opportunity to visit the National Medical Centre for Children in Washington DC and the National Children's Hospital of Pittsburgh, both in the USA, and the Hospital for Sick Children in Toronto, Canada. One of the main differences identified by the visit was the preparation for the role, as nurse practitioners in the USA have traditionally been prepared at graduate or Master's level since the development of the role in the late 1960s. Very few examples of ENPs, in the sense that they are known in the UK, were found, and the paediatric nurse practitioners undertook primary care and child health roles that would have been undertaken by our primary health care teams. Given that there are few, if any, American nursing qualifications that are comparable to those in the UK that lead to registration on Parts 15 and 8 of the UKCC register, the authors felt that they were able to confirm Jones' (1996) findings, namely that experienced children's nurses would make fitting ENPs if suitably trained and supported.

From protocols to practice

The next phase of the project was concerned with the development of protocols for practice for the envisaged categories of patients suitable for ENP management (see Figure 2.5). In order to identify those minor injuries and illnesses that might be suitable for nurse-led management, care protocols were developed with the medical and surgical consultants. A protocol has been defined by the RCN (1993) as 'an agreement to a particular sequence of activities that assist healthcare workers to respond consistently in complex areas of healthcare practice'.

For various reasons, the latter two categories in Figure 2.5 were never fully developed or implemented in practice. The nurses undertaking this roles were also able to prescribe 'one-off' doses of medication from a very limited formulary.

- Minor head injuries
- Minor wounds and abrasions
- Superficial scalds and burns
- Non-toxic poisoning episodes
- Mild asthma in children with a confirmed diagnosis
- Mild diarrhoea and vomiting

Figure 2.5 Categories of case for emergency nurse practitioner management

Delivering the training programme

Careful consideration was given to the content of the programme, and it was devised after consultation with professional colleagues who had developed similar programmes. The authors were mindful of the professional debate concerning the nature of advanced practitioner roles and acknowledged that the role of the ENP in this context could not be equated with that of the nurse practitioner graduates from the RCN nurse practitioner course or similar validated programmes of education. The curriculum and teaching and learning strategies identified for the course delivery were designed to reflect the needs of the adult learner and took the student's prior learning experiences and personal circumstances into account. The underlying philosophy was the need for children's nursing practice to be both evidence and research based (Glasper *et al.*, 1996), a variety of didactic and experiential learning activities being employed over the 5-day course that emphasised the development of the enquiring, reflective practitioner, based on advanced knowledge, skills and attitudes.

As well as the obvious subjects of applied anatomy and physiology relevant to the predicted caseload, sessions were also included on pharmacology and nurse prescribing; assessment and examination skills; the documentation of history and findings; legal and professional aspects of emergency care; paediatric and telephone triage; the practical management of patient categories and specific motor skills; and reflective journalling and critical incident analysis.

The teaching was undertaken by the authors and medical colleagues, who also supervised some aspects of the practical applications of theory to patient care. The aim was to enable experienced children's nurses to offer a service that complemented that of their medical colleagues, with the opportunity not only to lessen waiting time and increase patient satisfaction, but, more importantly, also to offer them a unique opportunity to make the best use of their knowledge, expertise and skills for the benefit of a specific client group. Additionally, they would be able to operate safely and professionally within clearly defined parameters and would acknowledge their responsibility and accountability for autonomous practice and clinical decision-making.

The management of children's minor injuries and illnesses in the A&E department

Wounds and abrasions

One of the most common reasons for a child to attend the A&E department is a minor wound or abrasion (Morton and Phillips, 1996), and care has to be taken that those wounds selected to be seen by the ENP are actually suitable for nurse-led management. Morton and Phillips enumerate the questions that must be asked in assessing minor wounds in children who present to A&E:

- Is primary suturing needed or advisable?
- Are deep structures involved?
- Is the wound free from foreign bodies and debris?
- Is the wound contaminated or dirty?
- Should this wound be managed in the A&E department?

The additional questions that begs to be asked is:

- Could this wound be managed by the children's ENP?

The protocol developed for the nurse-led management of children's minor wounds and abrasions was specific in the categories that could be seen by nurse practitioners and the classes of wound that should be excluded, the protocol having been developed in close collaboration with a consultant paediatric surgeon. The preparatory teaching for this care category had concentrated on the anatomy and physiology of the skin; the principles of wound healing; factors that might disrupt or delay healing; infection control and universal procedures; methods of wound closure; tetanus immunity; and the consideration of non-accidental injury.

An important aspect of the nursing role when caring for the child following minor trauma is that of health education and health promotion. It has been recognised that the majority of childhood accidents can be prevented and that the nurse in the A&E department is most likely to be involved in the tertiary aspects of accident prevention (Dearmun and Taylor, 1995), namely those of providing optimal treatment of injuries to ensure a complete recovery or to attempt to limit the amount of residual disability.

The nurse-led management of minor head injuries

The nurse management of minor head injuries would not appear to be commonplace, and to describe any injury as minor or trivial might be to disparage or denigrate the level of anxiety that parents may demonstrate when their child is ill or injured. In undertaking the nurse-led management of children's minor head injuries, there must be strict guidelines to ensure that serious injuries are not missed and that the mechanism of injury or the history does not preclude nurse management.

Head injuries account for about 10 per cent of children's attendance's at A&E departments (Morton and Phillips, 1996). Many of these injuries will be of a relatively 'trivial' nature and may well fall into the category suitable for ENP management, but it is important for there to be clear guidance on which cases may have complications and carry risks of secondary injury, or which may have been non-accidental.

Morton and Phillips (1996, pp. 93–4) offer sound and practical advice for taking a history and assessing the child with minor head trauma, and this guidance, together with the advice and expertise of paediatricians, formed the basis of the protocol used in Bristol. Again, the areas of health education and accident prevention are an important aspect of the nurse practitioner role, as is ensuring that the accompanying adults have a clear understanding and written and verbal confirmation of the reasons to bring the child back to the department, and of the home care and follow-up required.

Minor non-toxic ingestions

This protocol was written for children who had ingested a substance that was not sufficient either to cause harm or to require treatment. The nursing role is one of detective – to establish an accurate history of exactly what was taken when – and, again, to undertake parent education on the safe storage of medicines and household products.

Nurse prescribing

Nurse prescribing was initially recommended by the Cumberlege Report in 1986, but nurse prescribing is as yet still limited to the initial pilot sites in the community, despite evidence to show that nurses can prescribe effectively, economically and safely in all settings. The Royal Alexandra Hospital for Sick Children in Brighton recently demonstrated how robust protocols can be developed, thus satisfying the employing authority, which holds vicarious liability. The UKCC *Scope of Professional Practice* (1992, p. 8) states that:

> where it is the wish of the professional staff concerned, that practitioners in a particular setting be authorised to administer, on their own authority, certain medicines, provided that a local protocol has been agreed between medical practitioners, nurses and midwives and the pharmacist.

It may be likely that, in the future, children's nurses could establish a common formulary that would be useful in both the community and the acute setting, but until such a formulary exists, protocols may be a reasonable alternative, and, providing the nurse maintains accountability and responsibility, Brighton's example is a good one to follow.

- Paracetamol
- Ibuprofen
- Emla cream/Ametop cream
- Oral rehydration solution
- Histoacryl tissue adhesive
- Salbutamol

Figure 2.6 Useful medications for a paediatric prescribing protocol

Audit of practice

The audit findings of the first 10 months of ENP practice in the Bristol project confirmed that, in the cohort of 216 patients seen by the small numbers of ENPs (three full time and four part time), high levels of satisfaction were reported (Table 2.1). This concurred with national and international studies of nurse practitioner practice (Bowling and Stilwell, 1988; South Thames Regional Health Authority, 1994), namely that nurse practitioners offer care that is effective, safe and acceptable.

Table 2.1 Audit Results – Bristol, 1996

- ENP understood my child's needs – 94% total agreement
- ENP was interested in my child – 81% total agreement
- ENP seemed thorough – 86% agreement
- Less worried after seeing ENP – 74% (21% not worried in first place)
- Would follow advice given by ENP – 92%
- Came wanting to see ENP – 1% (wife of informant was a nurse practitioner)
- Came wanting to see doctor but saw ENP – 44.5%
- Didn't mind who saw child – 57%
- ENP gave adequate time for discussion – 97%
- Would want to see ENP again – 97%

The development of such a new service is almost certain to be limited to protocols and prescription of practice in order to promote safe practice and protect the public, although, as Cooper and Robb (1996) remind us, there are no nationally agreed parameters of practice. The very limited nature of the projected ENP caseload described in the Bristol project and the fact that it was protocol driven might lead some to question whether it was truly an expansion of children's nursing practice. Walsh (1989) contends that the nurse's role in this context can be so constrained by protocols and medical prescription that the notion of autonomous practice becomes almost meaningless. The role of the nurse practitioner is not solely defined by the range of tasks performed, nor by protocols or skill in diagnosis and treatment (Bowling and Stilwell, 1988). It encompasses the specific skills needed for practice but is underpinned by a philosophy of accountability for autonomous nursing practice.

In pushing forwards the boundaries of clinical practice, individual nurses must remember that they are accountable for their own actions and should not undertake new roles without adequate preparation and training. It is equally important that new roles are not developed at the expense of other aspects of nursing care or existing service provision. As Dimond (1996) points out, specialist areas of children's nursing practice should be closely scrutinised in relation to the UKCC's *Scope of Professional Practice* document (UKCC, 1992), and clear standards and areas of responsibility should exist.

The emergence of the children's ENP has evolved with the changing remit of the children's nurse and contemporary developments in the care of the sick child at home and in primary, secondary and tertiary care settings. The results of our preliminary audit, although informal, were highly gratifying but cannot be generalised to other settings or populations. The limitations that were encountered during the study were perhaps inevitable in a market-led economy of care, but, despite the fact that the role was disbanded when the authors both left the department, children's ENPs have the potential to benefit the working practice of all staff and, most importantly, to improve the care of children and their families.

However, such service developments must look beyond the mere expedition of care. Read *et al.* (1992), in a national survey of the role of the ENP in major A&E departments, concluded that, although such services are by no means the norm, there is great potential for the development of this role and practice domain. With or without nurse practitioners, the nursing role for children's nurses in A&E will continue to expand. Evidence exists to show that expanded nursing roles can enhance patient care in child health nursing, as demonstrated by the skill of inserting intravenous cannulae (Livesley, 1994). Many emergency nurses routinely perform expanded roles such as suturing, the application of plaster casts and so on, and it is the opinion of the authors that these 'tasks' are better performed by experienced and competent nursing staff within the holistic context of patient care than by junior doctors on short-term rotations.

In hindsight, the authors would have wished for the opportunity to have developed the training programme to an extent where it was validated by an appropriate educational body, not only to provide accreditation of learning, but also to defend their practice within the professional arena. As yet, there is no discrete educational provision for the preparation of child health nurse practitioners, although such programmes have long been offered in the

USA. This need is now clearly indicated given the fast-changing nature of health care demand and delivery, and the exciting developments in nursing practice.

A&E departments are the 'shop front' of acute care and are a vital link between the hospital and the community. The children's ENP of the future will need to be as conversant with the needs of the child and the family in the community as in the A&E department. We envisage that, in the future, children's nursing qualifications will be much better utilised in the A&E department, and our basic qualification prepares us very well for the development of ambulatory paediatric practice.

References

Audit Commission (1993) *Children First. A Study of Hospital Services.* (London: HMSO).

Audit Commission (1996) *By Accident or Design: Improving Emergency Care in Acute Hospitals.* (London: HMSO).

Bentley, J. (1995) Accident and emergency – still youthless? *Nursing Management,* 2(1): 22–3.

Bowling, A. and Stilwell, B. (1988) *The Nurse in Family Practice: Practice Nurses and Nurse Practitioners in Primary Care.* (London: Scutari Press).

British Paediatric Association (1988) *Joint Statement on Children's Attendances at Accident and Emergency Departments.* British Paediatric Association, British Association of Paediatric Surgeons & Casualty Surgeons Association. (London: BPA).

Burgess, K. (1992) A dynamic role that improves the service: combining triage and nurse practitioner roles. *Professional Nurse,* February: 301–3.

Cooper, M. and Robb, A. (1996) Nurse practitioners in A & E: a literature review. *Emergency Nurse,* 4(2): 19–22.

Dearmun, A.K. and Taylor, A. (1995) Nursing care of the child following minor trauma, in Carter, B. and Dearmun, A.K. (eds) *Child Health Care Nursing: Concepts, Theory and Practice.* (Oxford: Blackwell Scientific, pp. 507–8).

Department of Health (1991) *The Welfare of Children and Young People in Hospital.* (London: HMSO).

Dimond, B. (1996) *The Legal Aspects of Child Health Care.* (London: Mosby).

Dingwall, R. and Murray, T. (1983) Categorisation in A&E departments: 'good' patients, 'bad' patients and 'children'. *Sociology of Health and Illness,* 5(2): 127–48.

Glasper, E.A., Powell, C and Darbyshire, P. (1996) Children's nursing as a research based profession. *British Journal of Nursing,* 5(7): 420–1.

Hazinski, M.F. (1992) *Nursing Care of the Critically Ill Child.* (St Louis: Mosby Year Books).

James, M. and Pyrogos, N. (1989) Nurse practitioners in the A&E department. *Archives of Emergency Medicine,* 6: 241–6.

Jones, S.J. (1996) An action research investigation into the feasibility of experienced registered children's nurses (RSCNs) becoming emergency nurse practitioners (ENPs). *Journal of Clinical Nursing,* **5**: 13–21.

Jordan, S. (1993) Nurse practitioners: learning from the USA experience: a review of the literature. *Health and Social Care,* **2**: 173–85.

Kobran, M. and Pearce, S. (1991) The paediatric nurse practitioner. *Paediatric Nursing,* June: 11–14.

Livesley, J. (1994) Intravenous therapy – continuing education. *Paediatric Nursing,* **6**(4): 23–8.

Morris, F., Head, S. and Holkar, V. (1989) The nurse practitioner: help in clarifying clinical and educational activities in A&E departments *Health Trends,* **21**: 124–6.

Morton, R. and Phillips, B.M. (1996) *Accidents and Emergencies in Children,* 2nd edn. (Oxford: Oxford University Press).

Partridge, J. (1997) Environmental provisions for children in A&E. *Emergency Nurse,* **4**(4): 7–9.

Read, S.M., Jones, N.M.B. and Williams, B.T. (1992) Nurse practitioners in A&E: what do they do? *British Medical Journal,* **305**: 1466–70.

Royal College of Nursing IANE (1989) *Nurse Practitioners in Primary Health Care: Role Definitions.* (London: RCN).

Royal College of Nursing (1993) *Emergency Nurse Practitioners: Guidance from the RCN A&E Nursing Association and the Emergency Nurse Practitioners Special Interest Group.* (London: RCN).

Royal College of Nursing (1995) Protocols: guidance for good practice. *Nursing Standard,* **8**(8): 29.

Royal College of Nursing Children in A&E Special Interest Group (1995a) *Facilities in A&E Departments in the UK.* (London: RCN).

Royal College of Nursing Children in A&E Special Interest Group (1995b) *A&E Departments in the UK: Staffing and Annual Attendance Data.* (London: RCN).

Silver, H.K., Ford, L.C. and Day, L.N. (1968) The pediatric nurse-practitioner program: expanding the role of the nurse to provide increased health care for children. *Jama,* **204**(4): 298–302.

South West Thames Regional NHS Executive (1994) *Evaluation of Nurse Practitioner Pilot Projects: Summary Report.* (London: SWTRNHSE).

Stillwell, B. 1988) In Bowling, A. and Stillwell, B. (eds) *The Nurse in Family Practice.* (London: Scutari Press).

Thomas, D. (1992) Paediatric triage and assessment, in Budassi-Sheehy, S. (ed.) *Emergency Nursing: Principles and Practice.* (St Louis: Mosby Year Books).

UKCC (1992) *The Scope of Professional Practice.* (London: UKCC).

Walsh, M. (1989) The accident and emergency department and the nurse practitioner. *Nursing Standard,* **11**(4): 34–5.

3

TELENURSING – THE PROVISION OF INFORMATION BY TELEPHONE: THE IMPLICATIONS FOR PAEDIATRIC NURSING

E.A. Glasper and V. Wilkins

Castledine (1996), in highlighting the growth of paediatric nurse practitioners in North America, attributes their development to a shortage of doctors. Although nurse practitioner roles in North America are now underpinned by postgraduate Master's preparation, the emphasis has always focused on the enhancement of nursing assessment skills. Such skills are vital within the arena of ambulatory care, and there are a number of nurse-led initiatives related to telephone consultations that have developed into major research and development projects, telephone triage being one example.

What is telephone triage?

Triage, a common word in the nomenclature of nursing, is derived from the French word meaning 'to sort'. Traditionally used in an A&E setting to determine the urgency of intervention, the term is now being used in a variety of other settings where prioritisation of action, or advice, is the mainstay of management. One such area is in the growing field of telephone triage.

Telephone triage involves health care professionals such as nurses making decisions on a verbal history, often from fraught clients, and giving appropriate advice over the telephone (Glasper and McGrath, 1993). The type of advice that can be given by nurses during such a telephone conversation can fall into several areas (based on Knowles and Cummins, 1984):

- advice that prompts callers to seek immediate medical advice (this may be combined with verbal first aid instructions).
- advice that directs a caller to a health care professional, but with a lesser degree of urgency.
- advice that empowers callers towards self-care without the necessity of consulting a health care professional (at least in the immediate term or near future).
- information and advice-gathering.

It is the ability of nurses to deal effectively with clients seeking information over the telephone that has led to the development of sophisticated nurse-led telephone triage services in some countries, principally North America. Some hospitals, such as the Hospital for Sick Children, Toronto, Canada, offer in-service educational courses to equip telephone triage nurses with the necessary skills, knowledge and attitudes to operate such services.

In addition, the rapid changes in telephone technology, linked to a shift from tertiary to primary health care, have prompted the development of nurse-led telephone services. Furthermore, the emphasis on self-care and the growth in partnership with families has challenged children's nurses to dynamically extend their scope of practice. This has been fuelled in the UK by the UKCC's document *The Scope of Professional Practice* (UKCC, 1992), which has prompted nurses to re-evaluate their roles in health care provision. Late twentieth-century nursing now takes place in a variety of settings, not just hospital wards, and it is the field of ambulatory care that has diversified the practice of nursing. The growth area in which many nurses are becoming involved is the field of telephone consultations. This has been precipitated by an increase in demand by families for advice, information and counselling over the telephone. Despite this, there is a paucity of information related to telephone triage research within the UK. Innovatory work undertaken at the Royal Preston Hospital's A&E department has shown considerable demand for their service, but the service is non-dedicated, that is, nurses who answer telephones are also involved in the care and attention of ambulatory patients (Buckles and Carew-McColl, 1991).

Consumerism

The previous generation that remembered the austere times prior to the introduction of the UK National Health Service in 1947 was one which displayed few of the attributes of the modern consumer. On the whole, that generation were passive recipients of health care in an era when health professionals were benignly patriarchal, an era when a little information was thought to be dangerous. The establishment of the NHS was a great milestone in the evolution of health care because, for the first time, it became the right of every citizen to have a modicum of health care. Although the NHS is funded through taxation at source in the form of national insurance contributions, it is difficult for some people to grasp the reality that they pay for this service. The gratitude of the post-war population for the welfare state has ensured several generations of loyalty.

The growing consumerism of the 1970s, 80s and 90s is, however, beginning to affect the citizens' view of their personal health and the performance of their health service. The years of emphasis on tertiary mechanistic medicine to the detriment of primary health care is beginning to place a great strain on the fabric of the health service. As health consumers become more aware of treatment options in care and medical procedures, they have developed a sometimes insatiable appetite for information appertaining to their own or their families' health status. This appetite for knowledge has been exacerbated by the proliferation of the media, which has led to extensive coverage of health and medical issues on an almost daily basis. Health is very newsworthy, and some members of the Western population are now more health conscious than at any other time in history. This has led to consumers becoming more selective about health care and has accelerated the trend towards self-empowerment and thus self-care. Such elements of society now seek the necessary knowledge and support to stay healthy and to treat non-acute problems themselves. Because of this, some, although by no means all, families have fewer inhibitions in attending a family practitioner or a local A&E department.

Out-of-hours services

The increase in inappropriate out-of-hours calls upon family practitioner time is generating innovative methods of out-of-hours health care provision (Lattimer *et al.*, 1996). This has resulted from demand exceeding supply and situations in which some patients wait excessive periods of time to be seen by a health care professional. The use of a doctor's time in seeing non-urgent cases is proving to be a precursor to the concept of dealing with some patients using the telephone. It is recognised that the family practitioner is ideally placed to provide information to families.

However, Sharp *et al.* (1992) indicate otherwise, suggesting, at least in the area of psychosocial problems of childhood, that family doctors do not identify or manage them well. The growth in nurse-led ambulatory care clinics is indicative of the reality that, in practice, not every family doctor is able personally to offer every service demanded by patients and families. Although family practitioners do and can act as a health information resource for millions of families across the world, it must be appreciated that not all doctors receive consistent and thorough communications skills teaching during their pre- and post-graduate education. In addition, many family practitioners are overloaded with their existing workloads and are unable to consider taking on the additional responsibility of providing patient-orientated information services. Given that they can barely cope with the volume of clients presenting with acute medical problems, and that A&E departments are struggling to operate an efficient service, it is not surprising that there is a reluctance by some doctors to take an interest in anything other than clinical medical practice. If Castledine's (1996) assumption that the only difference in North America between nurses and doctors performing a primary care role is that nurses come from a 'caring educational base' and doctors from a 'curing base', it should be possible for a partnership that enhances patient care to develop between the two professional groups.

Family empowerment

The giving of information to families may be the key to their empowerment, and empowerment strategies are being pursued by children's nurses in an attempt to foster family-centred care. Thus family empowerment has become an integral component of advocacy (Brown *et al.*, 1996) and, as a consequence, has helped to shape some nurse-led telephone services, although it is yet to be rigorously tested through a randomised control trial. There is evidence that some groups in society are failing to take advantage of health services despite universal coverage. Flores *et al.* (1996) have shown that preventable morbidity and the underutilisation of health services can persist in high-risk populations, in this case native Americans. Flores and colleagues comment on similarities with the UK's NHS, pointing out that health services do not compensate for all the problems of social inequality or cultural barriers. The use of simpler, less expensive, focused preventative interventions might have a greater impact in preventing morbidity; these might include education, counselling, outreach and possible nurse-led telephone services.

Despite paediatric nursing's full adoption of strategic methods of empowerment and advocacy, there appear to be families who are unable to benefit fully from potentially therapeutic interventions. Miller (1987) has explored individuals' abilities to cope with stress and has provided a profile of some people who are information-seekers and others who are information-avoiders. This has important implications for those nurses who are attempting to give information to families by any method, in particular by telephone.

Telephone knowledge

Imparting nursing information to clients over the telephone is analogous to nursing with your eyes closed and your hands tied behind your back (Glasper, 1993). Because of this, nurses providing such a service require substantial specialised knowledge, skills and judgement (College of Nurses of Ontario, 1988) (Figure 3.1). This knowledge allows them to collect and analyse relevant data in order to determine the health needs of the caller and to recommend appropriate courses of action. Although it is recognised that telephone nurses require this type of educational preparation, there are no explicit UK directives in existence that advise nurses on how to provide such information to clients. The increased incidence of medical litigation will prompt the UK nursing profession to act swiftly, in order to address this situation effectively. Despite this, it is recognised that *The Scope of Professional Practice* (UKCC, 1992) addresses the extending role of nursing. The lack of specific guidelines related to telephone consultations is particularly worrying given that there has been an explosion in the provision of helplines over recent years, facilitated through the Health Services Guidelines document HSG 92(21), published in March 1992. Furthermore, the recently published UK government White Paper 'The New NHS' (1997) commits the Department of Health to providing 'NHS

Direct', a new 24-hour telephone advice line staffed by nurses for the whole of the country by the year 2000.

- Collaborate with appropriate health team members to establish policies, indicating who may provide telephone advice and under what circumstances
- Develop written guidelines to ensure that standard information is available. This will facilitate accountability and consistency of the advice
- Document each call received: a telephone log is a useful method. Documentation should include the date and time of the call, the caller's name, the caller's address, if not documented elsewhere, relevant data collected, any advice or information given and who handled the call
- Retain records according to the appropriate legislation
- Establish a mechanism for regular review of the guidelines to ensure relevance, accuracy and appropriateness of the information given

---

Figure 3.1 Guidelines for registered nurses providing telephone advice (College of Nurses of Ontario, 1988)

The increasing availability of helplines is leading to an exponential demand by health care consumers for such services. It must be highlighted that the existing UK regional health authority helplines that have developed since 1992 are usually operated by non-nurses and provide information of only a general nature. These helplines were launched by individual health regions to augment the concepts embodied within the original UK Patient's Charter (Department of Health, 1992), and these have been reinforced by the publication of the Children's Charter in 1996 (Department of Health, 1996).

A concern for the nursing profession is that the families or clients who contact these helplines may mistakenly believe that they can provide medical or nursing information. Given the disparate backgrounds of the individuals employed in running some helplines, the achievement of a homogenous service is impossible. It is for the nursing profession to appreciate that the Patient's and Children's Charters respectively, coupled with NHS reforms, have stimulated the purchasers of health care to explore new initiatives promoting client-orientated services. The development of nurse-led telephone triage may represent an example of how this philosophy enhances the drive towards patient empowerment that is so prominent within the two charters.

Telephone consultations

In some countries where information-giving to families and clients is more highly developed, nurses are recognised as playing a vital role in this field. Nurses are particularly good at developing skills to give information over the telephone. There is nothing particularly new about telephone consultations, and British health visitors have offered a service for many years to their clients, albeit on an *ad hoc* basis. British nurses have, however, been slow to respond to the challenge of improvements in the telecommunications industry, and at least one nurse has implicitly indicated that nurses should reacquire the lead in the development of telephone services for clients (McGrath, 1992).

Quilter Wheeler (1989) illuminates the embryonic stage of the development of telephone consultations and argues that telephone triage should be recognised as a clinical speciality in its own right. She believes that the nurse of the future, armed with a telephone and the appropriate educational training, can successfully avert crises within different patient groups. However, nurses will need to be proactive in developing their expertise within the overall field of telemedicine as there are other professional groups that are beginning to realise the enormous potential of telecommunications in the quest for patient and family empowerment. One such group that is extending its professional base is that of the pharmacists, who see themselves in a key role in the delivery of health information.

A recently launched freephone service in Toronto, Canada, entitled 'Pharmaplus' and run by pharmacists, is proving popular and has received considerable air time on local radio. Similar schemes are being considered for the UK, and the growth in such services should help to reinforce the necessity for nurses to respond to the opportunities provided by research in telenursing.

The telephone in Western society

The growth in telephone ownership since World War II has created an opportunity to use telecommunications technology as a vehicle to enhance quality health care. Newsome *et al.* (1996) reveal that 91 per cent of households in Great Britain have a telephone, representing a 49 per cent increase in ownership since 1972. Although there are regional variations in telephone ownership across the UK, the telephone has risen during the past 20 years from fifth to second place in the list of purchasing priorities, coming ahead of a washing machine.

Despite the increase in telephone ownership by members of the public, Hallam (1989) has highlighted that the number of general practitioner consultations by telephone has not risen accordingly. It is interesting to note that the first recorded telephone consultation in the UK occurred in 1879, when a doctor is reported to have used the telephone to discount the diagnosis of croup (Anon., 1879). Although much improved since 1879, the telephone is still regarded by many as simply a mechanism for relaying messages. Telephone communications between medical professionals is at an advanced level, but communication between a patient and a health professional has barely improved since the 1879 model. Although the use of the telephone in medical care is, therefore, as old as the telephone itself, it is the North Americans who have eagerly embraced its use. Despite this, the use of the telephone figures prominently in many health care settings. In particular, many family practitioner receptionists operate informal telephone triage services in an attempt to unravel the complexities of those clients seeking appointments.

Hallam, in her review of the use of the telephone in primary care, reveals that only 7 per cent of UK family practitioner encounters occur on the telephone, compared with 25 per cent in the USA. Rising costs of personal visits to family practitioners in the UK would suggest that an increase in the number of telephone consultations by physicians, nurses and other health professionals is inevitable. However, the use of the telephone by health care professionals is based on enthusiasm rather than research findings; Summersgill (1997) has highlighted the paucity of research and suggested that much of the existing evidence regarding telephone nursing is anecdotal.

Paediatric nurse-led telephone triage

Wilkins (1993) has described one of the world's few substantial telephone triage systems specifically designed for children and their families. The Toronto (Canada) Medical Information Centre, situated within the world famous 'Sick Kids' hospital, provides a 24-hour telephone advisory service for patients in metropolitan Toronto. In addition, the unit also provides a poison service for the province of Ontario. The telephone triage service in Toronto is staffed by 25 experienced nurses who possess a skill mix of clinical attributes, together with high-level communication expertise. The team of paediatric nurses alternates 12-hour shifts operating ten telephone lines. Ferguson (1992) gives a brief history of the Toronto Service, which began in 1977 with the aim of relieving the pressure on the 'Sick Kids' emergency department, which was being gradually inundated with telephone calls by worried parents.

Historically, parents in the metropolitan Toronto area have telephoned the Hospital for Sick Children seeking information or advice relating to their child's illness or injury. Prior to 1977, the hospital did not have a formal mechanism to respond to these questions (Taylor, 1992), and, as a result, parents may have been referred to any one of a number of health care professionals – a nurse, a pharmacist or a physician. These calls were not formally documented, nor did these health care professionals have protocols or policies to guide their practice. Without guidelines or the documentation of calls, it was impossible to ensure that the public received consistent recommendations from those responding to the public's queries.

In an effort to respond to the growing public demand for information over the telephone, the Hospital for Sick Children set up a telephone triage service entitled the Medical Information Centre (MIC) in March 1977. During this time, the hospital had received funding to set up a regional poison centre for the province of Ontario. The regional poison centre is also a telephone advisory service, receiving calls from the general public as well as health care professionals seeking advice on how to handle actual or potential toxic exposure. Nursing staff were selected to work in this new unit specifically to provide a telephone service for poison and medical information calls.

Documentation

Prior to taking calls, this group of nurses was responsible for developing unit policies, documentation forms and protocols. Protocols were developed following an extensive literature search and in consultation with specific medical specialists. The call volumes have subsequently increased from just over 1000 calls per month in 1977 to over 6000 calls per month in 1997. Parents in the metropolitan Toronto area indicate an overwhelming support for the service provided by this specialised group of nurses. Letters of appreciation from parents illustrate how effective such a service can be:

- The MIC line is an incredible lifeline for us, both practically and psychologically.
- The nurses are always extremely helpful, knowledgeable and calming/reassuring in their manner.
- I was able to get all the information from your helpline.
- As a result of contacting the MIC, we did not have to take our crying 20 month old into Emergency, but received enough information and reassurance to treat him at home until morning when we could see our family doctor.
- The MIC line was really there for us at a time when we felt abandoned.
- Fortunately none of my problems have been life threatening, but it is wonderful to have your service available. The response from your staff has always been intelligent, practical and sympathetic.

As with any inpatient chart, documentation is of prime importance. Every call received is documented, even if the person calling is looking for the answer to a simple question such as 'My co-worker's child has chicken pox. I work closely with this person; can I take the virus home and infect my children?' In order to obtain a complete and accurate history, the nurse must frequently be directive in her questioning as parents do not necessarily know what details are important. For example, a parent might telephone the MIC line requesting information on how to deal with a child who is vomiting; it is only through the nurse's questioning that the history of a head injury is obtained. Comments such as 'My child can't breathe' require further clarification. Is the mother describing a child who has a stuffy nose or a child who is experiencing inter-costal indrawing. The parent's 'sixth sense' or general impression of their perception of the severity of the child's illness is a worthwhile guide. Take seriously the mother or father who makes a statement such as 'I can't quite put my finger on it or describe it but my child just doesn't seem right.'

Auditing a random sample of charts is a small component of the telephone triage total quality management programme. Monthly random charts audits have assisted the Toronto team in identifying and correcting documentation inconsistencies as well as facilitating and identifying staff learning needs. However, it must be appreciated that there are cultural differences between Canada and the UK that may prohibit a wholesale adoption of the Canadian model.

Motherisk – a telephone service for mothers

The Hospital for Sick Children, in association with the University of Toronto, has continued the tradition of innovation within telephone consultations in launching the highly successful Motherisk programme. This telephone service has been developed to deal exclusively with pregnant and lactating women who have been exposed to potentially noxious compounds. The Motherisk telephone information service was inaugurated in 1986 and now deals with 30 enquiries a day for the province of Ontario, which has a population of nine million. The skilled telephone management of anxious mothers who may have ingested a hazardous material is a strong indicator of the future potential of this type of professional intervention.

Protocol development

Layton (1993) defines care protocols (also known as anticipated recovery pathways, collaborative care plans or critical pathways) as agreed interventions for a given diagnosis, symptom or procedure within a time limit. Protocols for telephone triage must be written by the multidisciplinary team, and their aim should be to focus the delivery of care on the patient and to ensure that the advice given is predictable and of a high quality. A continuing worry for paediatricians is when it is safe not to examine a sick infant. George *et al.* (1994) have discussed the ramifications of telephone consultations and recognised that the majority of such encounters will present no problems. It is the exceptions, such as the atypical presentation of meningitis, that are the real cause for concern for the telephone triage nurse. However, it must be stressed that concern over potential litigation need not inhibit the implementation of a telephone triage system. There have been no known cases of successful litigation in the nearly 20 years since the Hospital for Sick Children commenced its telephone triage service. Added reassurance of the competency of nurses to provide telephone advice is provided in a study by Yanovski *et al.* (1989). They have shown, in a study of telephone triage by family doctors in Philadelphia, that, during a simulation exercise, fewer than half of the surveyed group had obtained histories on the telephone that were considered sufficiently adequate to have ruled out potential serious illness. Dale *et al.* (1995) have discussed the development of a decision support computer software package as a method of improving nurse-led telephone consultations in an A&E department (a similar system is being developed at the Hospital for Sick Children, Toronto). The leap from paper-driven protocols to computer-generated interactive telephone protocols is thus already a component of the emerging discipline of telenursing.

Paley (1995) believes that clinical protocols offer many potential benefits for both patients and staff. He believes that the value of professional nursing in health care can be demonstrated in the development of protocols in all areas of nursing. This may be particularly true in the area of primary health care, where the role of nurses is particularly challenging. Lattimer and the Southampton team (1996) have examined the future provision of out-of-hours primary medical care and have shown that family practitioners are keen to try alternative arrangements for out-of-hours care delivery, including nurse-led telephone triage services, which they would be willing to pay for. Linking such new services to robust protocol development will undoubtedly enhance the quality of that service. Implicit within the telephone triage movement is the notion of self-care as this is a predominant feature of telephone management.

The dramatic increase in demand for out-of-hours primary medical care (Hallam, 1994) will place telephone triage in the spotlight of those initiatives which address and tackle the out-of-hours crisis. Some primary family practitioners have begun to exploit and augment the public's interest in self-care through the development of self-care protocols (Van der Does and Metz, 1993). It is suggested that families keep a dossier of self-care protocols by the telephone to remind them to ring the family practitioner only when necessary. Paediatric nurse-led telephone triage is beginning to lead the way in the development of family self-care, but its prosperity will be directly linked to the evidence generated from the ongoing research within the area.

Voice mail

The use of the telephone for health care is not restricted to the field of personal or family consultations. Although such telephone encounters between a professional and patient are developing in all Western countries, there remain many criticisms of this type of health care. Some of this criticism is related to the competence of nurses who provide such telephone advice, and physicians want to be reassured of their abilities. As a consequence, research activity must be directed at demonstrating the equivalence of a nurse-led telephone consultation with the outcomes of a family practitioner-led consultation. Recent innovations within the telecommunications industry itself are facilitating a more rapid utilisation of telephone triage. This is because some of the fears of medical practitioners are now less acute, as nurses operating such services can have access to medically qualified personnel through conference calls, fax machines, mobile telephones, personal computers, modems, the Internet and so on. The ability of nurses to have access to computer-held patient records will revolutionise telemedicine in the early years of the twenty-first century. There are, however, many clients who do not wish to consult with a health professional on the tele-phone, including those who simply want information related to a particular topic. The use of voice mail or pre-recorded health messages may address this need and allow callers access to a wide range of health-promoting strategies. The reduction in the cost of local phone calls (in some countries being completely free), coupled with the growing availability of subsidised 0800 free telephone numbers, makes voice mail an alternative option for health promoters/health educators.

The University of Wisconsin-Madison has led the way in the development of voice mail health care. The university's Health and Human Issues Division has created a tape library of health and medical information on an extensive range of subjects currently in excess of 600 topics. The so-called HEALTH-LINE is now being offered in many cities in North America, and a similar system is being offered by the Help for Health Trust, Highcroft, Winchester, UK. Winchester's Health Line, which was initiated in 1970, offers the caller a range of lay-orientated audio messages on such diverse topics as cancer and contraception. Each topical message lasts from 3 to 7 minutes. A subdivision of Health Line is Health Line Harmony, which offers a selection of more than 200 audiotaped messages focusing on child growth and development, and adolescent concerns. In addition, a further series of topics is designed especially for teenagers and young adults. Health Line works not by providing tapes *per se* to organisations, but by providing scripts that can easily be adapted for local use. Such a strategy allows sensitive cultural issues to be addressed. In addition, tapes can be recorded in a local dialect or using local nomenclature, thus giving a tailor-made feel to the initiatives.

Benefits of voice mail health promotion

- Patients or families can be prepared for medical procedures in advance, for example in how to prepare your child for hospital admission.
- Callers can get information on topics that interest them at any time of the day or night, for example a teenager wanting information on the drug Ecstasy.
- Health messages are a patient education resource. They can potentially release nursing time that might be otherwise spent in giving repetitive advice to clients.
- Callers appreciate the anonymity of the service.
- Callers can be helped to make informal decisions on a whole range of health matters.

The health services directorate of Health and Welfare, Canada, has conducted an exploratory study of health information and support telephone services in Canada (Romeder, 1993), initiated to provide documentation on these emerging telephone health information services. The study reinforces the notion that telephone services are becoming increasingly important to the general public in North America and that they appear to be an effective way of promoting health through the provision of information and support.

The majority of telephone health services have been introduced as development initiatives. Genuine research within the field to demonstrate potential outcomes is required because, without such robust research, it will be difficult to convince the potential purchasers of such services of their efficiency, particularly in periods of economic austerity. Traditional health promotion activities have concentrated on changing behaviour with a view to improving health. Romeder (1993) comments on the successes and failures of this approach and describes telephone health services as a health promotion strategy that is designed to improve individuals' abilities to cope with a health issue that affects them directly or someone close to them.

Education for telenursing

The provision of skilled nursing over the telephone requires more than experience and dedication. Robust educational programmes that are commensurate with the responsibilities of the telephone nurse are necessary to underpin the development of these services. The imaginative use of vignettes and role play allows novice telephone nurses the opportunity to rehearse typical and atypical calls. The development of telemedicine modules within Master's programmes will raise the status of telenursing overall.

Conclusion

Paediatric nurses operate in an increasingly technological age. They are being proactive in harnessing this technology to effect changes in their portfolio of empowering strategies. The utilisation of telephone triage, telephone helplines and telephone voice mail will allow paediatric nurses to provide families with the opportunity to learn more about their health or health-related problems. However, getting well or solving health problems is a two-way process, and callers to telephone services must play an active role (Tables 3.1 and 3.2).

Table 3.1 Nurse's responsibility during a telephone encounter

1. Being able to listen and gather information
2. Being knowledgeable about health and
3. Asking questions to gain relevant information
4. Giving information relevant to the problem in question or symptoms described
5. Asking the caller to decide what he or she will do about the problem, based on the exchange of information
6. Giving advice based on sound principles and stating when he or she does not agree with the caller
7. Documenting both the nursing assessment and agreed plan for future action
8. Telephoning the caller back if the nurse is uncomfortable about the outcome of the communication

(McGear and Sims, 1988)

Table 3.2 Caller's responsibility during a telephone encounter

1. Calling when he or she has a problem with, or a question about, his or her health
2. Giving accurate information about the problem
3. Being willing and prepared to answer any questions the nurse needs to ask in order to better assess particular needs
4. Listening to the information/advice provided by the nurse and asking questions if it is not understood
5. Deciding upon a course of action based on the information received and discussing this with the nurse
6. Contacting the service again if there is any change in symptoms or if there are further questions or problems

(McGear and Sims,1988)

References

Anonymous letter to the editor of the *Lancet*, 29 November 1879, p. 819.

Brown, D., Campbell, S., Glasper, E.A. and Glasper, J. (1996) Perusing strategies of patient empowerment – a preliminary evaluation of a CD-ROM generated health promoting information system. *Southampton Health Journal*, **12**(1): 18–21.

Buckles, E. and Carew-McColl, M. (1991) Triage by telephone. *Nursing Times*, **87**: 26–8.

Castledine, G. (1996) Extremes of the nurse practitioner role. *British Journal of Nursing*, **5**(9): 581.

College of Nurses of Ontario (1988) *Guidelines for Registered Nurses Providing Telephone Advice*. (Ontario: College of Nurses of Ontario).

Dale, J., Williams, S. and Crouch, R. (1995) Development of telephone advice in A&E: establishing the views of staff. *Nursing Standard*, **9**(21): 28–31.

Department of Health (1992) *The Patient's Charter*. (London: HMSO).

Department of Health (1996) *The Patient's Charter – Services for Children and Young People*. (London: HMSO).

Department of Health (1997) *The New NHS. Modern. Dependable*. (London: HMSO).

Ferguson, T. (1992) Caring for kids. *Imperial Oil Review*, 8–13.

Flores, G., Farrell, E., Rock, S.M., Cook, K., Morton, J. and Teel, J.L. (1996) Preventable paediatric hospitalisations and sub-optimal use of health services despite universal coverage. *Ambulatory Child Health*, **1**: 223–34.

George, S., Glasper, A., Hall, M., Long, G. and Newsome, C. (1994) Parental empowerment through clinical information. *Paediatric Nursing*, **6**(2): 11–14.

Glasper, A. (1993) Telephone triage: a step forward for nursing practice? *British Journal of Nursing*, **2**(2): 108–9.

Glasper, A. and McGrath, K. (1993) Telephone triage: extending practice. *Nursing Standard*, **7**(15): 34–6.

Hallam, L. (1989) You've got a lot to answer for, Mr Bell. A review of the use of the telephone in primary care. *Family Practitioner*, **6**: 47–57.

Hallam, L. (1994) Primary medical care outside normal working hours: review of published work. *British Medical Journal*, **308**: 249–53.

Knowles, P.J. and Cummins, R.O. (eds) (1984) Medical advice telephone calls: who calls and why? *Journal of Emergency Nursing*, **10**: 283–6.

Lattimer, V., Smith, H., Hungin, P., Glasper, A. and George, S. (1996) Future provision of out of hours primary medical care: a survey with two general practitioner research networks. *British Medical Journal*, **312**: 352–6.

Layton, A. (1993) Planning individual care with protocols. *Nursing Standard*, **8**(1): 32–4.

McGear, R. and Sims, J. (1988) *Telephone Triage and Management. A Nursing Process Approach.* (Philadelphia: W.B. Saunders).

McGrath, K. (1992) Close calls on the phone. *Practice Nurse*, October: 374–81.

Miller, S.M. (1987) Monitoring and blunting: validation of a questionnaire to assess types of information seeking under threat. *Journal of Personality and Social Psychology*, **52**(2): 345–53.

Newsome, C.A., Hall, M., Glasper, E.A., Long, G. and George, S. (1996) Telephone ownership: implications for the provision of health care and information. Unpublished manuscript, University of Southampton.

Paley, G. (1995) A framework for clinical protocols. *Nursing Standard*, **9**(21): 33–5.

Romeder, J.M. (1993) *Health Information and Support Telephone Services. An Exploratory Study.* (Ottowa: Health Services Systems Division).

Sharp, L., Pantell, R.M., Murphy, L.O. and Lewis, C.C. (1992) Psychosocial problems during child health supervision visits. Eliciting, then what? *Paediatrics*, **89**(4): 619–23.

Summersgill, P. (1997) Telephone triage: a panacea for child and family health care? *Journal of Child Health Care*, **1**: 11–16.

Taylor, W. (ed.) (1992) Baby you need this number. *Toronto Star*, 18 August.

UKCC (1992) *The Scope of Professional Practice.* (London: UKCC).

Van der Does, E. and Metz, R.G. (1993) *What Should I Do? Do I Go to the Doctor?* (Southampton: Dryden Brown).

Wheeler, S. Quilter (ed.) (1989) Telephone triage: lessons learned from unusual calls. *Journal of Emergency Nursing*, **15**(6): 481–7.

Wilkins, V. (1993) Paediatric hotline – meeting the needs of the community while conserving healthcare dollars. *Journal of Nursing Administration*, **23**(3): 268.

Yanovski, J.A., Malley, J.D., Brown, R.L and Balaban, D.J. (1989) Telephone triage by primary care physicians. *Paediatrics*, (4): 701–6.

4

DEVELOPING A CENTRE FOR HEALTH INFORMATION AND PROMOTION

E.A. Glasper and R. McWilliams

It has been argued that the key to family empowerment is the giving of information (Robertson, 1995). The success of ambulatory care in practice depends on high levels of communication with families. This stance is ratified throughout the UK Children's Charter (Department of Health, 1996), which identifies information-giving as a fundamental right of children and their families. Furthermore, Whiting (1997) has stated that children's nurses should focus their activities on the promotion of health rather than on sickness.

The message relating to the importance of information-giving is reiterated in the priorities and planning guidance for the UK National Health Service 1997/98 (NHS, 1996). This document, which is intended to produce an action response within the NHS, identifies that service users and their carers need a greater voice and greater influence in the overall management of their care. The document demands that strategic plans are developed and implemented to provide opportunities for families to become involved in their own care and to improve the quality of information and communication. This unequivocal directive from the UK Department of Health should produce a positive response among those health care professionals providing services to children and their families.

Despite this affirmation of the right to information, it is well known that the families of sick children hunger for ever-higher levels of information from health care professionals, and Bailey and Caldwell (1997) stress the importance of effective communication skills when giving information to families. However, there are some health care professionals who find it difficult to transmit to families what might be distressing news, and such individuals, in being benignly patriarchal, may withhold or dilute information when entering into a dialogue with families. The rapid memory degradation of verbally transmitted information makes it imperative that differing strategies of communication are developed which maximise technological innovations within the telecommunications industry, among others.

Although the UK Children's Charter gives a clear indication of what might be achieved within the area of family communication, it must be appreciated that many children's hospitals and units in a number of different countries have already implemented and developed those standards embodied within the charter. The gauntlet, having been thrown, has been picked up by many paediatric nurses working within the field of ambulatory care. Some of these nurses have demonstrated considerable imagination in the giving and sharing of information with families. Although the emphasis has been placed on giving information to parents/guardians, it must be appreciated that children themselves are often fundamentally disempowered through being denied access to information.

Alderson (1995) discusses the importance of giving information to children and highlights the need for written information to employ short lines, words, sentences and paragraphs. In addition, she argues that all aspects of communication with children, including Makaton and other sign languages, Braille and taped information, should be explored.

What is empowerment?

The term 'empowerment' has become somewhat of a buzz word in recent times, yet it is often misunderstood or used as a euphemism for any strategy that saves nursing time. The Collins 1987 English dictionary defines 'empowerment' as 'giving power or authority to, enabling, permitting'. The term stems from the Latin word *potere*, meaning to be able.

However, the rhetoric of empowerment is somewhat different from the concreteness of strategies of empowerment that purport to enable people to make health-related decisions. Although the pursuit of empowerment strategies by nurses is a recent phenomenon, it has become an integral component of advocacy. The term 'empowerment' is appealing because it conjures up images of power and independence. The nursing profession has embraced advocacy as a method of family-centred care, but the methods of achieving its implementation have changed considerably over the years. From a position of interceding or pleading a case for families, paediatric nurses are now acting as guardians for their rights to autonomy and free choice. Indeed, current health promotion ideology accepts empowerment as enabling and supporting people to set their own health agendas and to take control of their health status through skill development and critical consciousness-raising (Rodwell, 1996). Although many paediatric nurses have taken a proactive stance in the pursuit of family empowerment, some factors have impeded them from fully implementing such strategies. Chief among these factors has been a perceived loyalty to an employing institution, which may at times conflict with a loyalty to a patient. However, the move towards reflective practice identified by James and Clarke (1994) may allow nurses and other health care professionals to be more positive in representing their clients.

Although there have been many innovations in patient advocacy, and empowerment is a real force within the field of child care, it has to be stressed that patients and families are sometimes passive bystanders in the process and the resultant inequalities in the powerbase, that is, the health care professional–family relationship, can create a dichotomy between caring and empowerment (Malin and Teesdale, 1991). This point is stressed by Gann (1990), who applauds the emphasis on consumer-friendly services within the UK health service but is dubious about the sanctification of choice. Real choice is now the cornerstone of the British government's strategy for health care reform, and it is reassuring to see information provision figuring prominently in Patient's Charter standards. Nurse educators need to reflect this in curriculum design, and Rush (1997) believes that student nurses need the appropriate skills, knowledge and attitudes if they are to function in a health care setting that promotes family partnership.

A central tenet of Western governments' health promotion strategies, including the British Health of the Nation proposals (Department of Health, 1991) is to promote good health and well- being through health-promoting initiatives. Adams (1996) highlights that the principal aim of self-empowerment models of health education is to improve clients' health by developing their ability to understand and control their own health status. Although stressed as being important by inclusion in patients' charters, it is disappointing that patient information strategies are given little if any mention in hospital league tables. The failure to include this in, for example, the UK Hospital and Ambulance Service Comparative Performance Guide (Department of Health, 1994) is disappointing because the inclusion of information-giving would have encouraged a greater proliferation of such initiatives. The creation of hospital league tables may, however, be a precursor for an improvement in many areas of patient care and should not lightly be dismissed given that the underlying philosophy is to encourage a state of healthy competition between hospitals in which those with the poorest ratings will be motivated to achieve the standards of those with the highest ratings.

What is a centre for health information and promotion?

The primary aim of a centre for health information and promotion (CHIP) is to provide specialist informational material for carers and children to help them to understand and cope with health- and illness-related family concerns. Such family information centres differ from other types of health promotion units in that they are located within large tertiary hospitals and concentrate on families with sick children, although they also promote healthy lifestyles for all. A major role of any CHIP is to augment and support information provided by health care staff for families (Glasper *et al.*, 1995). The fundamental philosophy of a CHIP is to share complete and unbiased information with families in an appropriate and supportive manner. Steele and Willard (1989) believe that parents (and professionals) see the search for information as a positive way of coping with a new or difficult situation and see equal access to information as an integral part of a collaborative relationship. It is widely believed that the provision of information will enhance the relationship between the professional and the family, and it is this premise which underpins the growth of the CHIP movement.

Such an ethos underpins the Southampton Family Information Centre, which is part of the NDU situated within the children's outpatient department. The large variety of outpatient clinics offered within the department at Southampton, coupled with a busy A&E department, has generated an increased need for family-centred information and the promotion of family involvement in care. In addition, the shift of resources from tertiary to primary health care is encouraging hospitals to focus more broadly on health promotion. The provision of a CHIP within a busy ambulatory care area of a hospital allows nurses to become much more assertive in the promotion of health information and opportunistically involve even those families who in normal circumstances would prove passive in the pursuit of information.

Fundamental aims of a CHIP

1. To give parents/carers and children specific health information relating to health and illness, and treatments and care, provided by the hospital and/or community.
2. To co-ordinate and assure the quality, validity and reliability of all health information (written, audio or televisual multimedia) produced for children and their carers.
3. To develop information packages using appropriate technology for a wide range of situations and scenarios affecting sick children and their families.
4. To audit the usefulness and effectiveness of existing and new materials, in addition to keeping all materials current and up to date, reflecting equal opportunities and local community ethnic mix.
5. To respond to specific health concerns from patients, parents and families, and to serve as a referral source to health care professionals within and outside the hospital.
6. To promote health for all in responding to government guidelines instructions as appropriate.

The vast majority of parents want to understand what is happening to their children when they are ill or have a medical condition. Parents need to have this information if they are to give appropriate explanations to their children. Because children's concepts of health and illness change with age, it is generally acknowledged that sick children require explanations of illness explained in concrete terms. This is to prevent frightening fantasies of the effects of illness or distortions of medical knowledge (Eiser *et al.*, 1986).

CHIPs can employ a number of strategies through which they can achieve their aims:

- the organisation of materials that are designed to provide families with information appropriate to the care of children
- the promotion of partnership in care

- the creation of an infrastructure that allows all members of the multidisciplinary team to communicate with one another and individual families through the utilisation of appropriate technology, including the World Wide Web.

Although family information centres/CHIPS are designed primarily for families, they can and do act as an important resource for health care professionals working in all client settings. It must be appreciated that, in working with the families of sick children, nurses can actually empower themselves by improving their own knowledge base. Some CHIPs have been designed for specific client groups. The Parents and Professionals Resource Information Centre (PAPRICA) has been described by Miles (1996) as having a specific aim of assisting parents in a better understanding of the diagnosis of their child with a severe physical and learning difficulty. The simple concept behind the CHIP movement is to empower through information-giving.

Although the concept of information-giving is simple, it can in practice prove more complex. Generations of nurses have been educated within the framework of the nursing process, which emphasises the biomedical approach to health. Such an educational model is fundamentally reductionist. In order for nurses to embrace a health promotion perspective, they must adopt a more holistic approach to their nursing practice. Such an approach will promote a 'bottom-up' philosophy of health promotion.

Resourcing a centre for health information and promotion

Many centres around the world use a combination of staff with differing professional backgrounds. Nurses, play specialists and librarians are often complemented by volunteer staff because it is difficult in a world dominated by evidence-based care to provide an example based on concrete patient outcomes. Despite the financial austerity linked to the worldwide shrinking 'health care dollar', some nurses have raised sufficient sums of money to provide the infrastructure for a CHIP. It is the recurrent staffing costs that are the primary stumbling blocks to a continued service, hence the reliance on volunteers.

However, the use of volunteers, at least in countries such as the UK, is often poorly understood. Volunteers need to be valued in the same way as full-time professional staff and require the same amount of human resource investment as any other staff member. All too often volunteers are abused, thus preventing optimum service delivery. Changes in employment practice, early retirement, redundancy and so on have created a pool of well-educated people who genuinely wish to serve society in some way. This community resource can be harnessed and used to provide a far better range of service than would be possible with expensive salaried staff. It is important that careful consideration be given to the planning stages before placing an advertisement for a volunteer to assist in the running of a CHIP. The following points should be addressed:

1. What is the role of the volunteer – consult widely and develop a job and person specification.
2. Ensure that a full interview selection panel is convened. A police check will be necessary before an offer of employment can be made.
3. Volunteers will need to give an assurance that they are able to commit a specific amount of time to the position on a set day or days of the week (remember that volunteers must have holidays too).
4. In-service training for the post should be provided through an orientation programme.
5. A uniform should, where necessary, be provided, as should an appropriate identification badge.

Volunteers have been shown to work effectively with paid professional staff and make an enormous contribution to the provision of service for children and their families.

Some CHIPs, such as that located within the paediatric NDU at Southampton, have employed specific family information nurses whose specific brief is to co-ordinate and facilitate information for the families of sick children. Action for Sick Children (formerly NAWCH) in the UK, The Association for the Welfare of Child Health in Australia and The Association for the Care of Children's Health in North America, among others, have provided information to the families of sick children for many years, and the creation of CHIPs within children's hospitals owes much to their innovative flair for positive change.

Thompson (1994) has indicated that age-appropriate information and resources must be readily available for children and highlights the constant dilemma facing many children's nurses of where best to concentrate their efforts – the child or the parent. The reality is that they must do both, but it must be recognised that it will require special skills to prepare information for children of differing age groups. The indivisibility of the family as a unit belies the growing independence of children in Western societies and highlights the fact that many children are fundamentally disenfranchised. Despite the changing face of childhood in late-twentieth-century society, parents will continue to seek out information as a way of dealing with the problems of childhood. Coombes (1995) reports that 28 per cent of enquiries to the organisation Action for Sick Children are from parents wanting more information on preparing their children for hospital. Fradd (1994) states that if nurses are to empower families, they need to have gained empowerment themselves. The existence of children's nurses holding the title family information nurse can only enhance this trend. Nurses who have some library training coupled with excellent interpersonal skills with patients, parents, staff and members of the public may make good family information nurses. Given the nature of the information that may potentially be given to families, great sensitivity is required by any member of staff thus employed.

Locating a CHIP

Few individuals have the opportunity to build a family information centre in an ideal place of their choosing. Some hospitals, such as the Hospital For Sick Children, Toronto, have had the luxury of new buildings in which to plan their initiatives, but most organisations have to make do or adapt what space they already have – or do not have. CHIPs come in all shapes and sizes, some being merely a cupboard, others the size of a provincial library.

With the ideal location not always being available, planners have to consider what all retail outlets have as their priority, that is, accessibility and good signage or advertising. The Family Information Centre at Southampton, situated at the entrance to the ambulatory care area, was not in an ideal position because the corridor in which it was situated was also a busy thoroughfare to a tertiary regional neurological unit. Despite this, the planners employed a glass structure to give light and a feeling of space. Bright yellow plastic glazing bars were utilised to compliment the rainbow theme of the ambulatory care area.

All signage within the department utilises the rainbow theme, and block colours are used elsewhere to reflect the primary colours of the rainbow. The less than ideal position of the CHIP at Southampton heralded an opportunistic move to a more convenient position within 18 months of the opening. Fortunately, the money spent on building the centre was not wasted as it was subsequently converted to an ambulatory care adolescent centre. The new location is much preferable to the old in that the CHIP is now situated within the main waiting area of the ambulatory care unit. The design of any family facility should not be taken lightly, even if it is the size of a cupboard. The planning and design process should be multiprofessional and involve as many of the different users of the facility as possible. In designing a CHIP, nurses must learn to exert their influence on hospital planners who have so often in the past failed to involve nurses and other essential workers in the design of patient facilities. Carlyle (1993) reminds nurses that the participation of all potential users of a facility during planning and design is the best way to promote solutions that support caring. She further advises planners to focus in on what they want to do in a space rather than what they want to have in it. In this way, the focus should always be on the activities of the CHIP and the relationship between carers and children and families.

The range of services

CHIPs can offer a variety of services, and, while the focus is ambulatory care, they can provide an important resource for inpatient families. From traditional family information leaflets to sophisticated telephone helpline support, CHIPs are able to harness all innovations within the communications industry. The use of written information, audiotapes, 35 mm slides, videotapes, faxes, e-mail, the Internet, CD-ROM, voice mail and computer desktop publishing software can all enhance information-giving to families.

Pamphlets/leaflets/family information sheets

Simple information leaflets are most effective in the quest by nurses to empower families (Glasper and Burge, 1992). Many pre-written leaflets are available free of charge from a variety of agencies, for example the pharmaceutical industry, and government departments of health. However, pre-written leaflets are limited and are unlikely to satisfy all potential clients of the CHIP. Because of this, children's nurses may wish to develop their own; this is not difficult, although there are precautions which must be taken. Family information leaflets cannot just be keyboard generated one evening using the home desktop computer. Although they can be designed and easily produced using commercially available desktop publishing software, their contents require rather more skill. The use of experts to gather the information required for the production of the leaflet is mandatory, as is the necessity of piloting and field-testing of early prototypes.

Readability formulae

There are often assumptions made by writers of client information sheets that all will read and understand. In recent years, readability formulae have been employed by writers to assess patient education materials. Pichert and Elam (1985) point out that such readability formulae are not in themselves a universal panacea to correct the ills of a badly written piece of information. Despite this, the growth in the use of such formulae stems from health care workers' concerns relating to patients' abilities to read and comprehend instruction leaflets. The low level of literacy of some groups in Western societies is forcing some health care workers to adopt other strategies, such as the use of comic strips. Poor reading ages among other groups necessitate the use of simple, clear, and unambiguous language. Lang (1992) argues that all writers of patient information leaflets should:

- know their purpose (what they are trying to achieve)
- know their audience (whom they want to affect)
- know their subject (what they need to say)
- know the setting (the conditions in which their audience will read their text).

Patient information sheets have the advantage of being cheap and relatively easy to produce. They can be updated with little inconvenience and can project a corporate image for the department, unit or hospital. Their use in ambulatory care will undoubtedly continue to grow.

CD-ROM-generated information systems

Some CHIPs, such as the units within the Hospital for Sick Children in Toronto, and Southampton, have introduced CD-ROM-generated information systems. One such system is the Health Reference Centre on Infotrac, a CD-ROM source of information for many health-related topics. This CD is to a large extent a full text database of professional and lay health literature ranging from patient information sheets related to, for example, asthma to full academic medical papers from journals such as the *Lancet*. The system differs considerably from library-based CD-ROMs such as CINAHL and Medline in that the ability to access information that is organised by subject has been greatly simplified for patients, and the user may in most cases print the full paper rather than just the abstract.

In addition, this type of CD-ROM contains useful lay texts, including personal case studies and articles from popular contemporary journals and newspapers. Browne *et al.* (1996) have described a preliminary evaluation of a CD-ROM patient information system and have indicated support for its use among patients. The availability of professional staff for help in interpreting information received from such systems is clearly desirable, and the family information nurse can fulfil this role at a high level of competency. It is obvious that written computer-generated material and other methods of information-giving can never, nor should they, replace verbal explanations to families, but the adoption of differing strategies can only enhance good practice. In addition to CD-ROM systems, some centres are beginning to establish family information Internet Web sites where common information leaflets can be hung for the benefit of browsers. This method of information-giving is likely to grow as more people in the population gain access to the Internet.

Audiovisual information

When a family visits an ambulatory care facility, there are opportunities to expose that family to a wealth of health-promoting stimuli. Although a primary concern for the family will be the child's particular illness or condition, there exists a receptiveness to other health messages that can and should be exploited. Many children will visit a hospital outpatient unit before admission, and it is for this reason that some offer pre-admission material during the visit. Innovative units have produced videotapes explaining the hospital admission, whereas others use audiotape, slide or Internet programmes. The increasing availability of local and commercially produced audio-visual material suggests that it should figure prominently in CHIP planning. Strategically placed video/monitors may be used to promote a particular health message, particularly during the inevitable waiting periods that occur in all ambulatory care areas. It should be possible for CHIPs to play a vital role in the promotion of health generally. Particular campaigning, such as safe cycling, safe sunbathing and safe homes, is a particular feature of the Southampton unit (Lowson, 1995).

Evaluating CHIPS

The use of family satisfaction surveys, focused audits and other research tools is an essential component of the continued longevity of any ambulatory care facility. Units such as Southampton utilise a steering group to help the family information nurse plan her campaigns effectively. The involvement of a wider team in shaping the direction of the CHIPs cannot be overestimated. As ambulatory care becomes the cornerstone of a primary health care-led health service, it will be for the nurse-led CHIP movement to seize the opportunities thus presented for real improvements in family-centred care. The quest for research evidence to underpin the role of such units must continue, and children's nurses will need to publish their work in peer-reviewed journals to ensure that such evidence is widely disseminated among the profession. Without evidence, probable purchasers of such services are unlikely to invest in their development.

References

Adams, T. (1996) Voluntarism and health education in nursing. *British Journal of Nursing,* **5**(3): 153–73.

Alderson, P. (1995) *Listening to Children – Children, Ethics and Social Research.* (London: Barnardos).

Bailey, R. and Caldwell, C. (1997) Preparing parents for going home. *Paediatric Nursing,* **9**(4): 15–17.

Browne, D., Campbell, S., Glasper, E.A. and Glasper, J. (1996) Pursuing strategies of patient empowerment – a preliminary evaluation of a CD-ROM generated Health Promoting Information System. *Southampton Health Journal,* **12**: 38–43.

Carlyle, A. (1993) The impact of design on the caring environment. Unpublished paper presented at the 1st UK RCN Society of Paediatric International Nursing Conference. (University of Cambridge: Churchill College).

Coombes, R. (1995) From parent to expert. *Child Health*, 2(6): 237–40.

Department of Health (1991) *Health of the Nation*. (London: HMSO).

Department of Health (1994) *Hospital and Ambulance Services: Comparative Performance, 1993–94*. (London: Central Office of Information).

Department of Health (1996) *The Patient's Charter – Services for Children and Young People*. (London: DoH).

Eiser, C., Eiser, J. and Hunt, J. (1986) Developmental changes in analogies used to describe parts of the body – implications for communicating with sick children. *Child Health Care Development*, 12: 277–85.

Fradd, E. (1994) Power to the people. *Paediatric Nursing*, 6(3): 11–14.

Gann, R. (1990) Patient information. *Health Libraries Review* 7(4): 223–6.

Glasper, E.A., Lowson, S., Manger, R. and Philips, L. (1995) Developing a centre for health information and promotion. *British Journal of Nursing*, 4(12): 693–7.

Glasper, A. and Burge, D. (1992) Developing family information leaflets. *Nursing Standard*, 6(25): 24–7.

James, C.R. and Clarke, B.A. (1994) Reflective practice in nursing: issues and implication for nurse education. *Nurse Education Today*, 14: 82–90.

Lang, T.A. (1992) How to write patient education handouts. Unpublished document, Departments of Scientific Publications, The Cleveland Clinic Foundation, USA.

Lowson, S. (1995) The growth of an NDU in a paediatric outpatient department. *British Journal of Nursing*, 4(1): 36–8.

Malin, N. and Teesdale, K. (1991) Caring versus empowerment: consideration for nursing practice. *Journal of Advanced Nursing*, 16: 657–62.

Miles, G.A. (1996) Resource centre for parents and professionals. *Paediatric Nursing*, 8(6): 13–15.

NHS (1996) *NHS Priorities and Planning Guidance 1997/98*. (London: DoH).

Pichert, J.W. and Elam, P. (1988) Readability formulas may mislead you. *Patient Education and Counsellor*, 7: 181–91.

Robertson, R. (1995) The giving of information is the key to family empowerment. *British Journal of Nursing*, 4(12): 692.

Rodwell, C.M. (1996) An analysis of the concept of empowerment. *British Journal of Nursing*, 23(2): 305–13.

Rush, K.L. (1997) Health promotion ideology and nursing education. *Journal of Advanced Nursing*, 25: 1292–8.

Steele, B. and Willard, C. (1989) *Guidelines for Establishing a Family Resource Library*, 2nd edn. (Washington DC: Association for the Care of Children's Health).

Thompson, M.L. (1994) Information-seeking, coping and anxiety in school age children, anticipating surgery. *Children's Health Care*, 23(2): 87–97.

Whiting, L. (1997) Health promotion: the role of the children's nurse. *Paediatric Nursing*, 9(5): 6–7.

5

THE NDU AS A STRATEGY FOR CHANGE WITHIN AMBULATORY CARE

Susan Lowson and Stephen Wright

For us who nurse, our nursing is a thing
Which unless we are making progress
Every year, every month, every week,
Take my word for it we are going back

(Florence Nightingale, 1872)

This chapter illustrates an important example of how organisational change in a paediatric outpatient department has given the opportunity to a group of professionals to review their practice and work through a process of change. The aim was to establish a team, enhance working relationships, empower staff and improve practice. Empowerment of the nurses would, it was believed, create a more mature and professional approach, which would enhance clinical competence and foster greater confidence in the empowerment of families and patients (Lowson, 1995).

The purpose of a department must be clearly defined in terms of its business, its reason for existing and the special and specific contribution it might make to a wider system. The staff in the children's outpatient department (COPD) at Southampton believe that their families and patients have the right to the best professional care and attention at all times. The COPD is one of nine clinical areas in the paediatric unit and therefore competes for some resources (COPD, 1994).

In the current UK NHS, organisational culture is very powerful: it can both limit and improve effective health care delivery. NHS staff think and act in most parts of the UK as carers or support carers in hospital. Caring for others brings many stresses and strains, demanding that organisations must have in place both the will and the facilities to care for the carers (Snow and Willard, 1989). However, this caring culture is not yet present in every setting, reinforcing the difficulty that can be encountered when any change in practice is proposed. Phrases such as 'That's not my job', 'That's the way we do it here', 'I don't think that the doctors would like that' and 'We've tried that and it didn't work' are commonly heard in parts of hospital services when any suggestion of changing working norms is mooted. Resistance to change is a common phenomenon; many general managers and senior clinicians would like to know how to tackle the negative attitudes but feel impotent to do so. Many examples of effective change in clinical practice, such as that described by Pearson (1988) and Wright (1989), indicate that long-term, meaningful change is difficult if not impossible using 'top-down' methods, whereby managers and others seek to impose change. Alternative 'bottom-up' strategies, involving control of the change process by the staff at clinical level, appear to offer more fruitful ways forward.

Change also demands resources, not least in terms of time and money, if staff are not to carry the burden by themselves, for example being asked to do more on top of already full workloads. The resourcing of projects must also be a concern to any organisation that is to demonstrate that it has serious commitment to change. However, many 'flagship' hospital Trusts are reportedly seeing their once efficient departments slowly destroyed by government requirements for Trusts to make year-on-year efficiency savings (*Times*, 17 May, 1996). This may currently make staff even more apprehensive about change – it could mean their own post going, resulting in redundancy. However, this chapter will show how a process of change has produced a challenged and motivated team portraying confidence and professionalism in their manner and attitude (Koch, 1991). Despite the many difficulties that beset them, not least major organisational change in the wake of UK NHS reforms and budgetary constraints, they illustrate how it is possible to face these challenges and advance the quality of practice and relationships.

The appointment of a Senior Clinical Nurse (SCN) in 1992 to the paediatric unit had provided the opportunity to review nursing practice across the unit and also coincided with an opportunity to attend a meeting at the King's Fund Centre in London. The King's Fund Nursing Development Programme had been given the management responsibility of a grant (£3.2m) from the Department of Health

(England) to support the creation of more NDUs. Subsequently, the paediatric outpatients department was successful in applying for funds to implement change. NDU status, it was believed, was an appropriate medium through which to direct change in the environment, approach and culture of nursing in the paediatric outpatient setting. It needed to re-examine and advance its practices in the light of many organisations' changes, and current thinking and research in nursing in this speciality (Lowson *et al.*, 1992).

The grant was awarded to implement a more rapid implementation and evaluation of innovative practice. The work of some established NDUs in other specialities has illustrated that limited access to development monies slowed the rate of change. It was believed that modest sums (approximately £30 000 per unit per annum over a 3-year period) could accelerate and increase the effectiveness of the change process. Grants were commonly used, as in this case, to support additional staff development, contribute to the funding of new support posts and help fund research and project work (Salvage and Wright, 1995). The Southampton team won the full grant of £90 000 spread over 3 years.

Although the application had been completed by the SCN with the support of a paediatric member of University of Southampton's Nursing Studies Unit, the staff had, albeit apprehensively, been involved in the 'on-site' assessment by the King's Fund assessors. The team in the department had become used to conducting a routine of events daily and, as nurses, rarely used their clinical skills – many had worked in the department for many years. Some of the team had concerns over the reality of official NDU status, and some were sceptical that the innovations would never occur. Others, however, were hopeful and excited by the prospect of change. Commitment to change and innovation is an integral part of an NDU philosophy. Wright (1992) has described NDUs as 'centres of collaborative clinical change where nurses work together to achieve their goals and aspirations'.

In 1988, the King's Fund Centre set up the Nursing Development Programme under the leadership of Jane Salvage to foster the development of nursing practice. The centre is a charitable organisation committed to improving health and social care by supporting innovations and undertaking development work.

One of the imperatives behind the NDU programme has been to enhance the quality of care offered to patients and clients through the use of knowledge-based practice.

This chapter describes how the origins and development of change in the team through the sound education and preparation of individual team members have enabled them to achieve a steep learning curve and become comfortable with a cultural shift that has embraced their values, attitudes and behaviour. The key elements in transforming the culture and making the change have been:

- clarity of purpose, core values and objectives
- clinical leadership
- planned change.

A dialogue to clarify the purpose and direction of the NDU enabled the team to see their common goals and to set them in the wider context of direction within the directorate and the Trust. A steering group of multidisciplinary team members was set up to support the outpatient staff in considering their philosophy, core values and key objectives.

The steering group was chaired by the SCN, who was the designated clinical leader of the NDU. It is the role of the clinical leader in an NDU (Salvage and Wright, 1995) to ensure that continuous improvement is the norm and that, in this case, patient and family expectations of services would always be considered. The Director of Quality and Nursing for the NHS Trust was also a member of this group, not only for her expertise and influence in support of the NDU, but also as evidence of organisational commitment to the NDU – a defining factor of NDU status (Salvage and Wright, 1995). Additional members were three paediatric consultants and a range of the nursing and clerical staff from the department. Advice and support to the steering group came in from a project worker from the King's Fund.

A coherently planned change process was essential (Koch, 1991) to:

- reach all staff and involve them in our improvement aims
- educate everyone in the knowledge and skills for achieving improvement
- tailor the training to meet the needs of staff in terms of appropriateness, content and scheduling
- ensure that quality improvements were consistent with each other and going in the same direction
- facilitate or overcome predictable professional resistance to change based on fears of losing a skill, role or status.

To accommodate these, staff were encouraged to rewrite their job descriptions, reviewing their role in the department. An appraisal system was established to ensure that all members of staff were given the opportunity to develop themselves and their practice – an activity partly funded by the grant given to the NDU from the King's Fund. A combination of top-down and bottom-up approaches to change appeared to stimulate rapid change while generating a sense of ownership of the longer-term strategy.

As clinical leader of the NDU, the SCN was effectively the principal change agent. Broome (1990) defines a change agent as 'someone who identifies major problem areas, identifies the opportunity for change, builds a readiness and commitment, builds a renewing system through creating a climate for choice and establishes internal capacity to sustain the change effect to evaluate and review it'. The SCN therefore acted as a facilitator to the team, helping them to define and determine the process of change that emerged, and the team seemed comfortable with this. Being an experienced paediatric nurse with previous experience of working to effect change was an asset that aided the effectiveness of the role. It was, however, clearly recognised that the staff themselves were the experts in the outpatient environment and the roles needed to be openly negotiated. The clinical leader needed to support and facilitate them in building up a vision they wanted, creating a view of current performance, helping them to envisage new possibilities and develop a strategy for change that they felt comfortable with and could see as achievable.

The trigger factor in organisational change was considered to be the need for a change in the environment. Staff saw this initially as being the surroundings, furniture and so on, and an anticipation of possible improvements of this particular aspect of the NDU helped to create a sense that other things could also be changed by working together. For example, the staff decided to change from a traditional uniform into a more friendly outfit of polo shirt tops and navy trousers or skirts. In addition, the clinical leader considered it essential to facilitate shifts in agreement between organisational members concerning the goals of the department. It was vital for the team to gain ownership and their clarification of this new perception of ambulatory care was important in mobilising energy and enthusiasm to improve performance. Core beliefs regarding the purpose of the department needed to be addressed, and this was achieved through a family satisfaction survey completed in July 1994. This survey attempted to identify those factors that are genuinely important for those families who use the outpatient department. Eighteen families were interviewed in a semi-structured open-ended manner. The sample was recruited from different clinics, and an attempt was made to ensure variability in the same sample. The interviews were tape-recorded and analysed using thematic analysis. A large number of themes were identified by the steering group and were finally classified into seven topics:

- information and communication
- relationships and role
- rights and empowerment
- environment
- philosophy
- car parking and travel
- positive strokes.

These topics were then grouped together into a tentative model indicating the way in which each worked in relation to the other. The seven topics then became a framework for a questionnaire to a larger audience. A number of questions were asked, but two issues were most prominent. First, the sample had a very traditional and stereotypical view of the role and function of health professionals. Second, despite a large proportion of the sample being unable to identify a qualified nurse, the participants had clear views about what they expected them to do. These data and previous audits conducted in the department presented a good starting point for a series of working groups to deal with the issues that had been high-lighted.

The SCN, in facilitating the processes of change, required the skills of persistence and patience as the outpatient department team struggled with the complexity and difficulty of effecting the necessary changes. Persistence and patience are critically important at the difficult stage of breaking down the core beliefs of the old guard, getting new problems sensed and articulated in an organisation, developing a sense of concern that the problems are worthy of analytical and political attention, and then describing the new order, often through highly articulate and impressive visions of the future (Pettigrew, 1985).

NDUs are places where the 'contemporary ideology of nursing is put into action' (Pearson, 1988). Patient-centred care is a dominant theme in contemporary nursing ideology. Putting the family at the forefront and caring about their needs and desires has been a reflection of the enhanced development of the nurses' skills and the services they offer to families in the NDU. Attendance at study sessions and conferences, which helped to develop further skills and evaluation of practice among the nursing team, further stimulated the desire to improve services and push back the boundaries of practice. A team of people began to emerge who were empowered and enthusiastic in their work, able to see change as a challenge rather than a threat. Success in one area seemed to stimulate the desire for more change and action in others. This became evident as the atmosphere in the unit was transformed in line with the nurses' new- found confident, assertive and cheerful manner.

The concept of the named nurse standard in the Patient's Charter (Department of Health, 1991) has reinforced the view that the family should receive nursing care and support in the clinic environment. The role of the nurse in the ambulatory care NDU has been to identify that support. Staff have developed the use of a business card to enable families to contact their nurse following consultation. The nurses have become expert practitioners through working in their scheduled clinic and have developed their own status and role. This has occurred in the form of nurse-led clinics, for example a novel nurse-led approach to enuresis management (Phillips, 1995), and in others' expertise in special child health disciplines and being a 'regular' face for the family to connect with.

The introduction of formalised therapeutic play in the NDU has been an opportunity for the entire multidisciplinary team to learn new skills. The Patient's Charter indicates that relatives and friends of patients should be given information about the hospital and various conditions. This gave an opportunity for the development of a paediatric Centre for Health Information and Promotion (CHIP). The staff believe that the provision of family information will help parents in the care of their children and that this is essential in a family-centred environment because information-giving is the key to empowerment (Lowson et al., 1995). As a component of the NDU's work, these and other services are part of ongoing evaluation.

The project worker from the King's Fund assisted the NDU at regular meetings and, through telephone consultations, supported the team in their preparation for change. He suggested that change would be most effectively supported by planned programmes of personal and professional development, citing Martin's (1984) research recommending that creativity and change must be accompanied by:

- the presence of an effective nurse leader at clinical level
- positive management support
- the involvement of clinical staff in organisational decision-making
- opportunities for continued professional development
- the resources available and the suitability of the environment in which care takes place
- the values which they themselves hold about their client group, nursing and nurses.

Collectively agreeing and writing the department philosophy 'Families First' created a vision that was crucial to what followed – no longer was the physician the most important person in the environment; nurses had started to address the needs of their clients from their own nursing perspective.

While many dramatic changes took place in the quality of care for children and their families, and in the activities and relationships of the staff, the question has to be asked whether the organisation as a whole (that is, the NHS hospital Trust) benefited.

The hospital Trust has been able to refer to NDU status in the COPD in a very positive way – for a department at Southampton to be one of only 30 King's Fund-accredited NDUs in the country gives an immediate rise in status. The Director of Nursing and Quality has been a member of the Steering Group and, in the foreword for the *Second Annual Report*, wrote, 'It is with a sense of pride that I have observed a major cultural change in the COPD. The second year as a NDU has seen the growth of dedicated, competent and innovative nurses who are truly focused on ensuring that their patients and families receive the best possible care and attention at all times.' She concluded that she looked forward to 'continuing to work with such a well motivated team in ensuring that we achieve our "Vision for the Future"' (Hollingworth, 1995).

The ambulatory care team has been encouraged to share its plans and ideas by creating a describable and challenging vision of the future (Buchanan and Boddy, 1992). The change agent has been involved in attempts to 'sell' ideas and plans to other organisational members, using strategies that include open communication and participation as well as the sharing of information to ensure that the message is being conveyed. The Director of Nursing and the SCN have both undertaken these roles. In addition, all the NDU team have been involved in disseminating their work, both internally and at various professional conferences and other forums. Dissemination of work is also an essential defining criterion of an NDU (Salvage and Wright, 1995) in contributing to overall professional awareness of potential improvements in standards that can be taken up elsewhere. Raising the profile of the NDU in this way has contributed to the good standing of the Trust, both locally and nationally. Being seen to offer an excellent service is even more important than before in terms of the current trend towards market forces in health care.

Management education is the structured, formal learning process that often takes place in an institutional framework. Management development is the broader concept concerned with developing the individual rather than emphasising the learning of narrowly defined skills. It is a process involving the contribution of formal work experience (Smith et al., 1989). The Trust has further gained through the development of a highly skilled and motivated team in the NDU, which has spread its influence towards improving quality way beyond the narrow confines of the walls of the unit.

The team in the COPD have been given the opportunity to be at the forefront of the development of ambulatory care nursing practice. The unit has shown its commitment to the development of nurses and nursing practice. It provides an environment where nurses challenge normal practice in order to give research-based, improved care to families. Each nurse within the department has had the opportunity to develop a strategy for the introduction of new ideas.

Following completion of the project, there is a real sense of ownership by the team. Initially, the drive toward the NDU came very much from a small number of enthusiasts, but eventually the whole team increased their support and involvement. Ideally, the NDUs are clinically led by all the team from the start, but the reality of many practice settings is that there is often a need for a few enthusiasts who are motivated and able to set things in motion. For some units, more broadly based team support is something that may evolve over time as the change strategy unfolds (Salvage and Wright, 1995). There is no doubt that some staff were sceptical that the innovations would ever occur, but the clinical leader had to have initial vision to believe in them and the possibilities for developing the unit. The initial challenge, therefore, was to build a team of people who could TRUST, RESPECT and CARE about each other. The clinical leader had to use a participation management approach to organisational change to overcome resistance and win commitment to new ideas, similar to that described by Pettigrew (1985), who described this a 'truth, trust, love and collaborative approach to change'. Trust, respect and caring are the three essential ingredients of empowerment.

The nursing team has been empowered by an encouragement to develop the knowledge, attitudes and skills required for effectiveness in their current post and their career. This has in turn encouraged self-esteem and enabled the nursing staff to be assertive rather than aggressive. As mentioned in the initial paragraphs of this chapter, commitment to change and innovation is an integral part of the NDU philosophy, putting the family at the forefront and caring about their needs and desires. At the forefront of this change has been family-centred care, and, for the nurse to be effective, it has been essential for her to be equipped with the necessary skills and knowledge. Time and commitment spent on providing effective training has paid dividends in quality improvements in ambulatory care, and the nurses have been encouraged to develop strategies for empowering themselves, thus developing autonomy and authority to implement optimal patient care.

The challenge for all paediatric nurses involved in ambulatory care is to push forward the frontiers of nursing in order to achieve a real shift in emphasis that does justice to the concept of a primary health care-led service.

References

Broome, A. (1990) *Managing Change. Essentials of Nursing Management*, Ch. 4. (Basingstoke: Macmillan).

Buchanan, D. and Boddy, D. (1992) *The Expertise of the Change Agent*, Ch. 4 (London: Prentice-Hall).

COPD (1994) *Unit Philosophy.* (Department of Child Health, Southampton University Hospitals NHS Trust).

Department of Health (1991) *The Patient's Charter*. (London: HMSO).

Hollingworth, A. (1995) Foreword. Second COPD NDU Review. (Southampton: COPD).

Koch, H (1991) *Total Quality Management in Health Care*, Ch. 3. (London: Longman).

Lowson, S. (1995) The growth of an NDU in a paediatric outpatient department. *British Journal of Nursing*, **4**(l): 36–8.

Lowson, S., Glasper, A. and Campbell, S. (1992) Families first: the Southampton NDU. *Paediatric Nursing*, **4**(8): 6–9.

Lowson, S., Glasper, E.A., Manager, R. and Phillips, L. (1995) Developing a centre for health information and promotion. *British Journal of Nursing*, **4**(12): 693–7.

Martin, J.P. (1984) *Hospitals in Trouble*. (Oxford: Blackwell).

Pearson, A. (1988) *What are Nursing Development Units?* (London: King's Fund).

Pettigrew, A. (1985) *The Awakening Giant: Continuity and Change in ICI.* (Oxford: Basil Blackwell).

Phillips, L. (1995) Enuresis in children. *Nursing Times,* **91**(42).

Salvage, J. and Wright, S.G. (1995) *Nursing Development Units.* (Harrow: Scutari Press).

Smith, S.D., Pell, C., Jones, P., Sloman, N. and Blacknell, A. (1989) *Management Challenge for the 1990s: The Current Education, Training and Development Debate.* (Sheffield: Training Agency)

Snow, C. and Willard, P. (1989) *I'm Dying to Take Care of You.* (Redmond: Professional Counsellor Books).

Times (1996) Doctor condemns NHS Trust financing. *Times,* 17 May.

Wright, S. (1992) Exporting excellence. *Nursing Times,* **88**(39): 40–2.

Wright, S. and Salvage, H. (1995) *Nursing Development Units. A Force for Change,* Ch. 2. (London: Scutari Press).

6

THE VALUE OF PLAY IN AMBULATORY SETTINGS

Maureen Ballentine and Diane Gow

The chapter provides a brief theoretical context of play, as a backdrop to exploring the contribution of play in ambulatory settings. The therapeutic value of play is examined, as is the role it occupies in preparing children and their families for investigations, treatment and surgery. Specific consideration is given to techniques and strategies of distraction and relaxation, and examples of good practice are included. Current debates surrounding who should prepare children for day surgery and where this preparation should take place are presented.

History of playschemes in hospital

Play in hospital is an essentially post-war phenomenon. During the 1940s and 50s, experimental schemes were introduced at St Bartholomew's and St Thomas's Hospitals, London, but it was not until 1963 that Save the Children Fund Hospital Playscheme was established. The following two decades saw the implementation of 60 further such playschemes, the responsibility for which has more recently been devolved to NHS Trusts.

However, the case for hospital playschemes has still to be universally accepted. In 1989, Save the Children identified that fewer than half of the UK children's wards had paid play specialists and, in the report *Hospital, a Deprived Environment for Children?*, concluded that children in hospital need play provision, not only because they have a natural need to play, but also because of the special functions that play can fulfil for children in hospital who are in unusual, sometimes extraordinary and potentially threatening situations. The report concluded unequivocally that play provision should be available to all children in hospital. Failure to do so not only constitutes a neglect of their basic developmental needs, but also deprives them of the medium through which they can successfully cope with an experience of hospital.

The purposes of play

The term 'play' is applied to an ever-increasing range of behaviours in which children and adults engage. The importance of play has long attracted the attention of professionals from many fields of study (Petrillo and Sanger, 1980; Rodin, 1983; Bolig, 1984) and is usually categorised in an attempt to understand its many facets.

Theories of the purpose of play began to emerge in the late nineteenth century, in particular from Spenser, Croos and Hall, but it is from the work of Piaget and Freud that much of the current understanding of children's play has been derived (Save the Children, 1989).

Play now occupies a prominent position in all spheres of child health. It is widely recognised to be crucial to the child's development in a variety of domains: physical, intellectual, linguistic, emotional and social.

Play allows children to adapt to the needs of their own culture. Through play, a child can learn about developing relationships with others, to learn to share, to take the role of leader or follower in a group, to learn to take turns, to feel in control of a situation and to respect other people's feelings. Play can be a spontaneous activity or something that can be planned in advance.

The planning can often give as much pleasure as the actual activity. It can be stimulating, allowing the natural curiosity of the child to be aroused, or a relaxing pastime. It can allow a child to make choices and to be in control, and it can be rewarding. An aspect that is rarely referred to in literature is that it should also be fun.

Play assists the child's development in a variety of ways. It provides the child with opportunities to develop a mastery of self and the environment, and test reality; it can be used as an outlet for needs and wants that may not otherwise be expressed. It provides a mechanism for dealing with fears, fantasises and emotions in a safe place and secure environment, thus providing children with the opportunity to master specific anxieties that cannot be resolved realistically. It can fulfil wishes and transform passivity into activity (D'Antonio, 1984; Bolig, 1984; Vessey, 1990).

Therapeutic value of play

For the child in the home environment, play constitutes a substantive part of daily life, and a child will usually need little prompting to play in a way that gives enjoyment. In contrast, children in hospital are likely to dealing with novel and peculiar stress related to injury, illness or treatment. They may be hesitant to play and may require assistance. Through giving children permission to play and by providing play equipment, we can help to overcome some of these barriers. Play in this context provides a crucial sense of normality for the child, and indeed the family, by allowing them to do something they know well. By encouraging other family members to enjoy and interact in the activity, anxiety can also be reduced.

When staff join in with the play, the therapeutic relationship is enhanced and the child will often be able to co-operate with staff. Play therapy, in all its forms, can facilitate a smoother adjustment and transition to the new and potentially frightening surroundings that the hospital environment poses.

Play in A&E departments

The A&E department is often the child's first experience of hospital. While some children may appear to be only mildly apprehensive about this encounter, for others it may be a desperately unhappy and frightening experience. If children's knowledge and understanding is indeed based on their life experiences, this can be very limited when a child first attends an A&E department. Conversely, it may be very vivid if a previous traumatic experience has occurred.

Unfamiliarity, combined with pain and bewilderment, will make it extremely difficult for the child to comprehend the situation in which he finds himself. It is therefore vital that the nurse is sensitive to the needs of the child and family, and is able to communicate with them.

The circumstances in which a child is taken to A&E confer little or no opportunity to prepare the child. Thus the need for appropriate explanation in brief, simple, clear and honest terms is paramount in terms of helping the child to come to terms with what will happen. Indeed, Eiser (1990) found that children who are not well prepared and are subject to invasive procedures show increased verbal and physical aggression, behavioural regression and greater anxiety.

Also, in the same way as adults, children suffer from loss of autonomy when they enter the hospital environment. Involving them in decision-making will provide a sense of control that should mitigate some of their situational anxiety.

The child may require treatment that is likely to be invasive, painful and distressing. In anticipation of this, a number of strategies are available to allay or minimise some of the distressing aspects of treatment. Techniques outlined by Lansdown (1987) focus on helping children to cope with needles; the principles are, however, applicable to many treatments that may be perceived as threatening to a child.

The techniques embody the following principles. The first is distraction, whereby, by focusing the mind on something other than the procedure, a barrier can be formed between the body and the mind (a process based on wartime evidence of soldiers in combat often sustaining serious wounds without feeling anything until they returned to base). Second comes relaxation, wherein the more relaxed the body, the more the sensation of pain is reduced (a principle enshrined in childbirth classes).

Distraction

Distraction is a seemingly simple but powerful approach, in which a variety of methods can be used. These include:

- singing and stroking, for the very young child
- counting – children could be asked to count as high as they can, or given an object with something to count on it; it may help if an adult counts with the child
- mathematical puzzles, doing sums in their head or counting backwards from 100 in threes, with the added distraction of the adult deliberately making mistakes for the child to notice
- jokes, for example, 'knock knock' jokes in which the child has to pay attention in order to join in
- blowing bubbles and the use of games such as noughts and crosses
- computer games, videos and personal stereo
- story-telling – making one up especially for the occasion, which has the advantage of being fresh and, if well told, will hold the child's attention while he or she is waiting to find out what happens next. The child may wish to join in with the story as it progresses.

The timing of distraction is all important. If commenced too early, the focus has gone before the needle appears or investigations or treatments are commenced. If started too late, the child may already be in a heightened state of anxiety, in which case more time needs to be spent with the child working through his or her fears in order that the child can regain some choice and control of the situation, that is, by renegotiating the timing with the medical staff in order to spend more time establishing the child's coping mechanisms. This is a powerful example of advocacy in practice. The nurse can involve children in some elements of choice, such as whether they want to look, asking them whose lap they would like to sit on and spending time revisiting relaxation and distraction strategies. Children may be upset that they have been perceived as naughty, and they will need reassurance that it is all right to be upset by these things. An arrangement can be made with the children, however, on how they wish to vent such feelings.

The parents are also in need of considerable support. They may be encountering feelings of helplessness, distress or embarrassment. It may be valuable to ensure the family are not feeling overcrowded and intimidated, asking any excess staff to leave to create some space for the family to gain some equilibrium.

Relaxation

The most common principle of inducing relaxation is to encourage the tensing of muscles in sequence, followed by a rapid relaxation of that muscle. One method is as follows. The child squeezes an adult's hand, breathes in and tenses his or her body while the adult counts to five. The adult models this by squeezing back and being tense at the same time. The position is held for 2 seconds, and, slowly counting from five to one, the adult gradually relaxes the child's hand while the child breathes out. This sequence should be repeated a couple of times before the procedure, then, for example, breathing in as the skin is cleaned and breathing out as the needle goes in.

Post-procedural play is also beneficial to enable the child to work through the experience. This may include drawing a representation of what happened, using teddies or dolls to depict the scenario.

There is much that can be done to achieve a more child-focused environment in A&E. If a dedicated children's A&E department is not in operation, there should be a separate waiting area for children and young people (NAWCH, 1987). This should be appropriately decorated and equipped with a range of play activities (see below).

Parental needs

Parents accompanying their child to the A&E department are likely to be fraught and anxious, which has been suggested to potentiate further anxiety in the child; this is known as the emotional contagion effect (Glasper and Thompson, 1993). They may be contending with a variety of overwhelming concerns for their child's best interests and how they may be perceived as parents.

Parents in distress may be pressing home to the child that the injury has occurred because the child did not follow their advice or instruction. While this may be true, it only serves to reinforce the potential for the child to view unpleasant treatment as a punishment for the 'wrongdoing'. Parental reactions may be centred on how the accident could have been avoided, while parents of a sick child may feel that they should have recognised their child's deteriorating condition earlier. They may encounter feelings of inadequacy as parents. Anxiety is exacerbated by ambiguity and uncertainty, a particular feature of waiting in A&E departments. This has been shown to hamper the ability clearly to appraise events, and limits coping (Mishel, 1983). When uncertainty is apparent, information may be distorted.

An important function that parents expect professionals to fulfil is that of clarifying uncertainty and providing answers. Nurses appear to occupy the important role of advocate and intermediary in these circumstances. Concern about unknown outcomes may be so consuming that it hampers the parents' ability to support and reassure their child (Rodin, 1983; Hogg, 1990). Through patient listening and reassurance, and the updating of developments via unambiguous information, the nurse can allay some of these feelings and thereby help parents to concentrate on the present and reassure their child (Ley, 1991). Parents should be encouraged to rehearse any questions they may wish to ask and write them down in advance of the consultation. As outlined by Visintainer and Wolfer (1975), giving accurate information about events, procedures and role expectations enables the child and family to cope more effectively with the various stresses encountered in a hospital experience.

In addition, parents may be accompanied by their other children, as alternative arrangements are difficult to achieve at such short notice. Therefore, supervised play areas help to reduce the intensity of the atmosphere and accommodate waiting times. If organised sensitively, this can help to reduce situational anxiety and distract children from the potentially distressing sights and sounds frequently associated with A&E (Hogg, 1990).

Play activities could include soothing media such as rice and sand. Imaginary play can take place in a home corner or a road corner, or using transport games. Dressing-up clothes such as child-size doctors' and nurses' outfits can be made available. Construction play and card games can be highly absorbing. Children's painting and drawing can sometimes be quite revealing in terms of their perceptions of what is happening.

The location of the play area is important: it should be in full view of parents and staff, to ensure adequate safety supervision and to overcome potential problems or parents' reluctance to go into the play area for fear of missing their name being called. Equally, the children will need to be able to see their parents at all times.

Outpatients department

This may be the child's first planned visit to hospital, either as a patient or as an accompanying sibling. This has special significance in terms of creating first impressions and realising the potential for a positive experience.

Play services in this area cater for a variety of needs. These range from keeping high-spirited children well occupied, by channelling their natural energies, through to taking referrals for children who are to be admitted.

Thus a full range of toys and activities should be available in this area. If possible, adolescents should have their own waiting area and all their appointments at a specified point in the day. Particular facilities for adolescents may include a television and selection of videos, music, computers, table football, snooker, craft activities, cards and boxed games.

For younger children, play materials could include construction equipment such as Meccano or Lego. Clay, sewing materials, puzzles, books and magazines can be of value. The main play area should include messy play activities. Trays of rice or pasta are relaxing and can be supplemented with sieves, spoons and water wheels. Supervision is needed particularly for glueing activities, collage, painting, playdough, sand and water play. A home corner with imaginative play materials including dressing-up clothes, dolls, cars and drawing is naturally engaging for the child and can help the parents to relax.

Play is usually interrupted for consultations or tests. Wherever possible, sensitive closure to the play should be achieved or it can be arranged that the child can take the activity with him or her to avoid unnecessary frustration and upheaval. Following the consultation, parents should be encouraged to allow their child to finish playing before removing them from the area, thus ending the visit on a positive note.

Children may be required to undergo tests and procedures in the outpatients department that are potentially distressing, such as skin pricks for allergy testing. Distraction techniques for such procedures can be invaluable. These include blowing bubbles for younger children, playing with small toys, searching for objects or people hidden in pictures and playing music quietly. Similar techniques may be used for taking blood samples and may include controlled breathing techniques (see above).

Children may be required to go on to other areas for tests such as X-rays, nuclear studies or ECGs. Where possible, play materials should be taken with them if they are not routinely available, especially as it is likely that children will have to wait to be seen. Children visiting other health professionals, such as the dietitian, can be encouraged to make pictures or collages of food and drink to reinforce the information given.

Regrettably, not all children have designated children's outpatients departments but are seen in adult or joint clinics, where peer grouping is particularly important and the environment needs to be adapted sensitively and appropriately in terms of decorations and equipment.

Outpatients may also be the department in which parents and children are informed of the need for admission. This is likely to arouse fears and anxieties that are best dealt with at an early stage. Play specialists should be available to take referrals of children who are to be admitted. Advice can be given on how and when to prepare the child for admission. However, Harris, cited by Glasper (1993), found that, in a study of 60 children admitted for a short stay in a paediatric ward for elective surgery, nearly half of the parents had received no explanation from the consultant at the initial outpatient visit. Most of the parents had no idea what would happen to their child in hospital, and most did not ask. The main reason given for not asking was the perception of the consultants' lack of time, exemplified by the queue of people waiting to be seen. Many hospitals recognise this paradox and rely on mailed literature as the vehicle for preparing parents and children for hospital, although pre-admission leaflets vary enormously in quality. While pre-operative information is now widely accepted as a useful tool in mitigating pre-operative anxiety, its use in child health has still not been fully exploited. Examples of high-quality information are found in Thornes' *Just for the Day* (1991). Ideally, literature should be provided for the child to understand and enjoy. It can include hospital stories, colouring cards and activity books for younger children. Information needs for children with a long-term illness who are likely to be attending frequently for day treatment should not be overlooked.

Essentially, information leaflets should cover general issues, procedures, the outpatients proforma, post-operative information sheets and the discharge letter and instructions, and individual visits can be arranged after outpatients visits.

If no pre-admission programme is established or time for a visit is not available, an album of photographs covering admission procedure, anaesthesia and the ward itself is a useful last-minute alternative.

Children's concepts of hospitalisation

Eiser (1984), in her review of preparation for hospitalisation, found that it was difficult to isolate any individual aspect of care that was especially helpful. The only consistent positive finding appears to be attempts to improve communication with children.

In order to be able to give appropriately tailored information about events, procedures, sensations and role expectations, there needs to be some understanding of the potential threats perceived by children in hospital and their developmental concepts of illness.

A study undertaken by Visintainer and Wolfer (1975) identified the features of hospital that can be a source of anxiety for a child. The following categories emerged, each of which has implications for the management and preparation of children undergoing (treatment) surgery:

- physical harm or bodily injury in the form of discomfort, pain mutilation or death
- separation from parents and the absence of trusted adults, especially for pre-schoolchildren

- the strange, the unknown and the possibility of surprise
- uncertainty about limits and expected acceptable behaviour
- a relative loss of control, autonomy and competence.

Interestingly, Visintainer and Wolfer quote evidence showing that the more emotionally upset the patient, the more medication is required, the more difficult it is for the patient to take drinks and the longer it takes for them to pass urine post-operatively (an important physical parameter for determining fitness for discharge following day surgery).

Children under 6 years of age had significantly higher manifest 'upset ratings', showing significantly less co-operation than older ones, although it has been argued that older children would be less likely to show their distress in such obvious ways (Muller *et al.*, 1992).

Whatever the precise interpretation of the results, however, one finding remains clear: the experience of hospital is, to varying degrees, a stressful one for children.

Preparation for day surgery

Play therapy provides an opportunity for children to understand and master their treatment which is unequalled by other preparation. (Eiser, 1990, p. 22)

With the information provided by more than 40 years of cumulative data, practitioners clearly recognise that hospitalisation is an inherently stressful experience for children and their families. Thus the momentum to care for children in their own homes and for hospital stays to be kept to a minimum has been high.

While brief isolated hospitalisation may be considered to be less traumatic, hospitalisation must nevertheless still be considered a crisis, as both opportunity and danger exist for coping, adaptation and continued learning. Even on a day case basis, hospitals still have many characteristics that can cause unprepared children to be frightened. Within a 24-hour period, children will still meet a large number of different people who attend them and to whom they are expected to relate. They may find themselves in a strange environment where it is hard for them to predict anything. As day cases, they will sleep in a different bed and will be given different food and different clothes, such as hospital gowns. In addition, they may be subjected to upsetting, confusing and often painful medical procedures, and the very people they have come to trust and rely upon look as worried and confused as they are themselves (Muller *et al.*, 1992). While improved paediatric care has undoubtedly reduced the risk of adverse effects for children undergoing occasional or short admissions, the possibility of long-term, serious sequelae remain for some (Eiser, 1990). The risk is greater for those experiencing frequent admissions, including children with chronic illness.

If the previous encounter has been an unhappy one, it is likely to precipitate a negative reaction, particularly where surgery has been experienced. Therefore the nature of the previous hospitalisation is significant in terms of adverse or positive previous separations and experiences of hospital. There is a need to be sensitive to other stressful experiences prior to day surgery. The emotional state of the child before admission has been suggested to be the single most important factor associated with disturbance resulting from hospitalisation (Brain and Maclay, 1968). The proposed timing of elective surgery may be influenced by issues such as the recent birth of a sibling, the death of a pet, a move to a new house or a new or first school.

Who should prepare?

The preparation of the family for impending admission and discharge should be mandatory if the full benefits of day surgery are to be realised (Glasper, 1993), yet few health authorities have established programmes to do this. It would appear that while health care Trusts pursue day care policy, what is often absent is investment in pre-operative, pre-admission information-giving. The Audit Commission (1993) suggests that many units demonstrate a lack of vision and an absence of policies, objectives and operational guidelines. This is consistent with conclusions reached by Azarnoff and Woody (1981) over a decade ago, who discovered that the preparation of children for hospitalisation was all too frequently left to common sense.

Preparation in schools

It has been suggested that preparation for hospital should feature as part of a wider general education. Elser (1989) argues that the classroom can be a valuable place to teach young children about hospitals and health care. This is an important arena for helping children to be prepared to deal with the adaptive tasks associated with a hospital admission and to develop coping skills and skills of seeking information.

Basic awareness of bodily parts could be taught in primary schools, for example giving outlines of bodily parts and being asked to draw or label certain organs. Talks by hospital staff on what they do is valuable. (In a similar fashion, children already have visits from firemen, police and road safety officers.)

School-based programmes tend to adopt one of three approaches. Hospital tours may be used, in which the emphasis is on familiarising the child with the local hospital. Alternatively, the hospital may come to the child. Muller et al. (1992) described schemes whereby play hospitals are set up in schools and children are given the opportunity to play with equipment. Other schemes have attempted to create a mini-hospital wherein scenarios were developed by hospital staff to represent admissions, radiology, surgery and special care. Hospital staff describe to children what happens at each of the five scenes, with ample opportunity for play with volunteers from the hospital. Children who took part in this programme showed fewer medical fears and had improved medical knowledge compared with those who did not participate (Muller, 1992).

Videos can make an important contribution to preparing children for hospital, although there are potential dangers if videos are shown to groups of children with no provision to answer questions as they are arise. They should be seen as a starting point of adequate preparation rather than an end in themselves.

Glasper (1993) highlights the benefits of outreach visits, a system commonly used in the USA and Canada, wherein hospitals liaise with their local nursery schools to provide teachers and children with information about local paediatric services.

Although in the UK Action for Sick Children became involved in school-wide preparatory programmes, their involvement was discontinued in 1982 when James Robertson, as a member of NAWCH, expressed concern regarding the danger of unnecessarily arousing anxiety in young children concerning separation, bodily mutilation and the pain of operations. He endorsed preparation information only for those children with planned medical or surgical procedures.

Hospital-based pre-admission programmes

Many hospitals now offer a variety of intervention programmes to familiarise children with hospital and treatment. The aim remains to reduce associated fear and anxiety. It has been suggested that preparation has been aimed primarily at children about to undergo short-term surgery. Rather less attention has been given to the needs of chronically sick children undergoing repeated and painful procedures.

Principally, such pre-admission programmes in the UK are undertaken on paediatric wards or units where the children will be admitted, in order to orientate families and prepare them for forthcoming hospitalisation. They may comprise a period of free play, using hospital-orientated toys, such as nurses' and doctors' clothes, theatre hats and masks. The use of skilled play specialists is essential in pre-admission preparation as they are best placed to address any misconceptions that the child may have about coming into hospital. The role of the children's nurse is also unique in terms of providing a complementary role in the quest for understanding through play.

Specific procedures-related play equipment may be used to prepare children for venepuncture; these may include jigsaws and activity books, which depict aspects of having blood samples taken. Rodin's study (1983) elicited three important findings in this area. First, children using these materials exhibited less anxiety during blood tests than those who did not. Second, anxiety was found to be further reduced for those children who had also been prepared by their parents. Third, there was also a direct link between parental anxiety and that of the child.

Firmly embodied in most pre-admission programmes is the use of films and narrative slide presentations covering aspects of the hospital stay from admission to discharge. An evaluative study by Bowlby, cited by Glasper (1993), revealed that children exposed to a preparatory film showed less disturbance post-operatively, made an earlier recovery, returned to school sooner and achieved higher parent satisfaction rates than did those of families in control groups.

A number of programmes incorporate a tour of relevant clinical areas, including a visit to operating theatres, where families can be orientated and clarification of issues regarding parental access can be provided.

Such play schemes may conflict with parental views if they do not wish their children to know why they are coming into hospital or indeed that they are coming in at all. Such a protective response is not uncommon, but every effort should be made to try to convince parents that fear of the unknown must be worse than being told in a kind and truthful way about what is likely to happen. There are profound and far-reaching implications for violating a child's trust when mistruths are perpetuated:

Children always come to some conclusions on their own whenever information is withheld. These are usually erroneous and painful. (Petrillo and Sanger, 1980)

The parental role in shaping a child's response is crucial, and their involvement in preparing their child for a hospital experiences is paramount. The onus remains upon hospital staff, however, to ensure that parents are furnished with the necessary prerequisite knowledge and information to feel more confident in preparing their child and to be able to answer questions as they arise. Early studies by Vernon (1965) found that lack of information was a prime cause of anxiety and that anxious parents were less able to provide the support and a sense of security for their children at a time of stress. Indeed, Ley (1991) proposed that the more a parent is prepared, the less is their situational anxiety. Mishel (1983), in her doctoral thesis, emphasised the importance of giving clear, comprehensive, and consistent information, having found that ambiguous information hampers the ability to appraise events and limits coping.

Parents should therefore be encouraged to be present throughout the day of admission, with written information provided in advance to prepare them for the responsible role they undertake. Leaflets should be in non-technical, user-friendly language, consideration being given to translating them into the languages of local minority groups.

Thornes' (1991) valuable report *Just for the Day* proposes that literature that addresses general aspects of day case admissions should include a leaflet covering general aspects of day case admission, a description of the ward and regular procedures, including:

- ward atmosphere and appearance
- ward routines
- the need for parents to plan journeys to and from the hospital, including the instruction that two adults are needed if one is driving the car
- the preparation of the child

- organising the family
- what to bring for the child and parent
- where to report and how to get to the ward (including a map or plan of the hospital, highlighting parking, admission location and refreshments)
- the role of the parent
- pre-operative procedures on the ward (for example, the use of topical local anaesthetic cream, whether premedication is usual, and, if so, whether a choice of injection or oral medication is given)
- anaesthetic, theatre and recovery procedures
- post-operative care on the ward
- probable discharge time and what happens if the child is not ready
- sources of information and discharge advice
- tips on travelling with a child who has had a general anaesthetic
- facilities for parents and young siblings
- general information about making arrangements for the child to be at home for the few days following the admission
- some idea of how support will be provided once the child has been discharged.

Communicating with children

Characteristics of thought at different ages appear to influence children's concepts of illness and therapy. This has significance in terms of explanations offered to children relating to their treatments and investigations.

Much of our understanding to date in this area has been influenced by the view of Piaget. Although subject to a number of criticisms, it has been the basis for a number of other enquiries in this field (Petrillo and Sanger, 1980; Bibace and Walsh, 1980).

The Piagetian view of children's cognitive development would propose that children aged 3–6 years have characteristically egotistical thinking, believing that the world revolves around them, with events happening because of their actions. Thus they readily perceive illness and hospitalisation as punishment, and have a propensity to fantasise. Bibace and Wallace have suggested that children between the ages of 2 and 6 are often unable to reason beyond the present and their immediate environment. Explanations have to be related to immediate cues. Tomorrow could be light years away for the distressed 2-year-old, and mummy going could be forever. Thus when explaining issues concerning time, it may be valuable to use concrete, familiar parameters such as mealtimes, a parent coming home from work and so on.

Speece and Brent (1984) suggest that children under the age of 7 may also have difficulty grasping the concept of reversibility and may consequently be unable to visualise awakening from anaesthesia. They also tend to categorise; thus if a child's relative has died after an operation, all operations may represent death. Gellert (1962) has proposed that many 4–6-year-olds appear to believe that all their bodily parts are indispensable.

Some of these concepts can be explored with the child through drawing and painting. For example, when a child drew what he perceived would happen in relation to an endoscopy, he thought he would be left with a big mouth, and a child awaiting tonsillectomy depicted himself on the operating table, his head had been taken off to remove the tonsils as they were not visible to the eye.

It should be noted, however, that providing children with the opportunity to explore these issues through play does not necessarily mean that they will spontaneously do so. Play may be a natural activity to children, but in an unfamiliar and threatening environment they can simply withdraw and regress. In such circumstances, children may need to be helped to play, particularly with the contribution of the play specialist who is able to provide considerable insights and strategies in a variety of domains.

Other mechanisms for explaining treatment include the use of a calico doll, which has been shown to be highly beneficial (Mathews and Silk, 1992). It can be transformed to demonstrate intravenous infusions or traction, for example. It is possible to insert bags of coloured solution attached to cannulae via plastic tubing so the child can actually draw 'blood' (coloured water) out of the doll. The child can also give injections and simulate skin testing and other procedures on the doll. It can be drawn on by the child to tell us how it feels and where it hurts, and drawn on by the adult to explain what is going to happen and how we can make it feel better.

Preparing children for X-rays and related radiographic investigations warrants special attention. Referring to an X-ray machine as a camera may be misleading. A child will not have encountered a camera of such large and daunting proportions. Having prepared children with respect to the size of the equipment, they need to be reassured that although it will move up and down and round, it is fixed and safe at all times and will not touch them. Being tipped up on the X-ray table may be likened to being on a fairground ride and a CT scan to being in a spaceship. In nuclear medicine departments, it is likely that the child will need an injection of radioactive isotope and a series of radiographs while keeping very still for 20 seconds or more. Following the application of a local anaesthetic, an explanation should be given to prepare children that the needle may sting. To help the child to keep still, he or she may wish to practise this with an adult. Being distracted with balloons, music tapes and musical toys can very effective.

The use of visual imagery can be valuable for young children undergoing lung function tests once they have had time to be acquainted with the equipment, for example by asking them to imagine they are blowing up a car tyre or blowing the rain clouds away. However, when communicating with children, the use of metaphors can be confusing and frightening if not used carefully. Swanwick (1990) uses the example of lungs being described as balloons, which may, of course, go off bang.

Conclusion

As has been seen, play can help children to resolve stress and conflicts arising from stressful situations associated with hospital experiences. As such, the value of playschemes in hospital has been established beyond refutation, but good practice in this domain is spread unevenly across the UK. This could be rectified in part by the introduction of hospital play specialists and facilities for play in every area that caters for children. The challenge for scarce resources cannot, of course, be ignored, but such provision does not necessarily require additional funding. Instead, it is a case of establishing proper priorities within existing budgets. The impact that hospital play has been shown to make on the quality of the child's experience of hospital places it squarely on a high priority agenda (Save the Children, 1989).

References

Audit Commission (1993) *Children First. A Study of Hospital Services.* (London: HMSO).

Azarnoff, P. and Woody, P. (1981) Preparation of children for hospitalisation in acute care hospitals in the United States. *Paediatrics*, **69**(3): 361–8.

Beattie, R. (1994) Animal magic. *Nursery World*, 7 April: 16–17.

Bibace, R. and Walsh, M. (1980) Development of children's concepts of illness. *Paediatrics*, **66**: 912–17.

Bolig, R. (1984) Play in hospital settings. In Yawkey, T.D. and Pellegrini, A.D. (eds) *Child's Play: Developmental and Applied.* (Hillsdale, N.J.: Lawrence Erlbaum.

Brain, D. and Maclay, I. (1968) Controlled study of mothers and children in hospital. *British Medical Journal*, **1**: 278–80.

D'Antonio, I. (1984) Therapeutic use of play in hospitals. *Nursing Clinics of North America*, **19**(2): 351–9.

Eiser, C. (1984) Communicating with sick and hospitalised children. *Journal of Psychology and Psychiatry*, **25**: 181–9.

Eiser, C. and Hanson, L. (1989) Preparing children for hospital – a school-based intervention. *The Professional Nurse*, March: 297–300.

Eiser, C. (1990) *Chronic Childhood Disease*. (Cambridge: Cambridge University Press).

Gellert, E. (1962) Children's conceptions of the content and functions of the human body. *Genetic Psychology Monographs*, **65**: 293–411.

Glasper, A. (1993) *Preparing Children for Hospital Admission. An Evaluation of Southampton's Preadmission Programme*. (Southampton: University of Southampton).

Glasper, A. and Thompson, M. (1993) *Advances in Health Nursing*. (London: Scutari Press).

Harris, P.J. (1981) Preparation of parents and their children for a planned hospital admission. *Nursing Times*, **77**(42): 1744–6.

Hogg, C. (1990) *Play in Hospital*. Play in Hospital Liaison Committee.

Lansdown, R. (1987) *Helping Children Cope with Needles*. (London: Department of Psychological Medicine, The Hospital for Sick Children, Great Ormond Street).

Ley, P. (1991) *Communicating with Patients*. (London: Chapman & Hall).

Mathews, M. and Silk, G. (1992) *Young Children, Priority One*. (Melbourne, Australia: Kwanis).

Mishel, M. (1983) Parents' perception of uncertainty concerning their hospitalised child. *Nursing Research*, **32**(6): 324.

Muller, D.J., Harris, P.J. and Wattley, L. (1992) *Nursing Children, Psychology, Research and Practice*, 2nd edn. (London: Chapman & Hall).

NAWCH (1987) *The Emotional Needs of Children Undergoing Surgery*. (London: NAWCH).

Petrillo, M. and Sanger, S. (1980) *Emotional Care of Hospitalised Children. An Environmental Approach*, 2nd edn. (Philadelphia: J.B. Lippincott).

Rodin, J. (1983) *Will This Hurt?* (London: Royal College of Nursing).

Save the Children (1989) *Hospital, a Deprived Environment for Children? The Case for Hospital Playschemes*. (London: Save the Children).

Speece, M.W. and Brent, S.B. (1984) Children's understanding of death. *Child Development*, **55**: 1671–86.

Swanwick, M. (1990) Knowledge and control. *Paediatric Nursing*, June: 18.

Thornes, R. (1991) *Just for the Day*. (London: NAWCH).

Vernon, D. (1965) *The Psychological Responses of Children to Hospitalisation and Illness. A Review of the Literature*. (Springfield, IL: Charles C. Thomas).

Vessey, J. (1990) Therapeutic play and the hospitalised child. *Journal of Paediatric Nursing*, **5**(5): 328.

Visintainer, M. and Wolfer, J. (1975) Psychological preparation for surgical patients. *Pediatrics*, **56**: 187–202.

7

PAEDIATRIC ONCOLOGY AMBULATORY CARE

Louise Hooker and Sarah Palmer

Childhood cancer affects approximately 1 in 600 children under the age of 15 years; each year around 1500 children in the UK are diagnosed with the disease, the most common form being leukaemia, followed by brain tumours. Advances in treatment can now offer cure in 60–70 per cent of cases. This has been achieved through centralisation of care, the development of intensive multimodal therapy and improvement in supportive care.

Childhood cancer is recognised as a chronic life-threatening condition and, despite improved prognosis, exerts an immense practical and psychological burden on the child and family over many years. The paediatric oncology ambulatory care setting provides families with expert medical and nursing care throughout the course of the illness, whether that means into adulthood as a long-term survivor or to the child's death. Very little published research is available within the area of paediatric oncology ambulatory care. The pathways lie open to important and exciting areas of research as many advances and developments may exist. This chapter aims to explore contemporary issues relevant to this very specialised care setting, the physical aspects of the ambulatory care facility, the importance of family education, and issues surrounding the documentation of nursing care and developing paediatric nursing practice.

Introduction

The provision of ambulatory care in the paediatric oncology setting has developed dramatically in the past decade and presents nurses with a double challenge: professionally, to support and provide nursing care to children and their families throughout treatment;

and practically, to ensure that technical medical procedures are performed efficiently and safely (Brenner, 1994). Nurses are now taking an active role in all aspects of treatment, providing not only practical care, but also education, support and friendship to the child and parents throughout their cancer experience (Reams, 1990).

Full spectrum of care

The day care setting in paediatric oncology exists to provide care to the child and family in an educational, supportive and counselling capacity in addition to the traditional therapeutic and practical role. Day care spans the complete spectrum of treatment from pre-diagnosis to terminal care and bereavement counselling.

Reaching diagnosis

A number of tests, investigations and procedures are often neces-sary in order to reach a diagnosis. This often involves preparation directed towards these procedures. The nursing staff or specifically trained play specialists can assist, using photographs, pictures, games and hospital play equipment to aid preparation. In nearly all cases, children are admitted as inpatients while investigations aimed at reaching a diagnosis are carried out.

Treatment

Cancer treatment can involve one or a combination of chemo-therapy, radiotherapy or surgery (multimodal therapy). These can be carried out as an inpatient or an outpatient depending on the situation, the child's condition, the treatment involved and the type of cancer.

Clinical review and supportive care

Routine clinical examinations, blood tests and investigations are an essential part of cancer care both for children on treatment and for those who have completed treatment. They are important for moni-toring the child's response to cancer treatment, the side-effects of the drugs and other therapies, and the early detection of recurrence or relapse of the disease. The supportive care for side-effects caused by treatment is often managed as an outpatient, that is, blood or platelet transfusions or the symptomatic control of pain or nausea and vomiting.

Long-term follow-up clinic

Patients who have completed treatment and are being reviewed every 6 months or annually attend a long-term follow-up clinic. Although the child or young person may feel essentially well and is to all intents and purposes cured, it is important to monitor any long-term side-effects of treatment, considering their physical, emotional and social well-being. Depending on the malignancy they had and type of treatment they received, specific investigations are undertaken, for example of hormone function for growth and development, cardiac function, renal function, fertility or secondary malignancy (Kissen and Wallace, 1995), and for any problems in readjusting back into society after their treatment for cancer (Eiser and Havermans, 1994). It is also important for clinicians, nurses and all professionals to see some of the survivors of childhood malignancy.

Palliative care

When no further curative treatments are available, families and hospital staff try to work out a plan that will provide the best quality of life for the child, usually with a minimal number of hospital visits and more supportive community care (see below).

Support groups

Some centres have set up different groups to cater for the needs of different individuals in similar situations, for example:

- therapeutic playgroups, for outpatients as well as inpatients and siblings
- teenage support group for patients

- sibling support groups, for children whose brother or sister is receiving treatment
- parent support groups, for parents with children receiving treatment
- sibling bereavement groups
- parent bereavement groups.

Care by telephone

Much of the organisation and delivery of care takes place when the patient is not physically in the hospital; nurse–patient contact is by telephone (Nail *et al.*, 1989). This may be initiated by nurses 'following up' patients at home to assess potential problems and provide support, or by families telephoning with concerns. It is important that care provided in this way is recognised as 'nursing by telephone', and staffing levels must also reflect the demands represented by the nursing needs of patients outside the ambulatory care unit. To ensure that nurses' skills are utilised effectively, clerical staff are needed to answer the telephone, deal with purely administrative queries and refer callers to nursing staff appropriately.

Physical layout

The actual location of a paediatric oncology day care unit can often be restricted by the physical limitations and facilities available within the hospital setting. Indeed, some hospitals treat their oncology inpatients within general paediatric wards; others are fortunate enough to have specialised paediatric oncology wards. Day care can take place in a general outpatient department, which could potentially be a risk to the children's health as they are often immunocompromised as a side-effect of their treatment. It is preferable that ambulatory care is managed in the same location as the inpatient treatment on a purpose-built paediatric oncology unit. This allows outpatient treatment to become an integral part of total care, minimising the fragmentation for patients and families and increasing the nurses' role in the holistic approach to paediatric oncology (Reams, 1990).

Oncology ambulatory care requires a fully staffed and well-equipped unit. A combined in- and outpatient unit allows for joint facilities such as treatment areas, a playroom, kitchen facilities, a parents' room and consultation rooms for all health professionals to use with families. Most large centres have a treatment area where children can be anaesthetised for lumbar punctures and bone marrow aspirates within the unit itself; this is easily managed on an outpatient basis, but it is a labour-intensive procedure and adequate numbers of appropriately trained staff are therefore necessary. Nurses must be able to assess, plan, document and evaluate the nursing care of patients during these invasive procedures (NHS Managment Executive, 1993). Nurses must also develop skills in the management of children's medical fears, behavioural coping patterns and pain perception during procedures (Broome, 1994).

A combined unit allows an easier transition from inpatient to outpatient care for the family and continuity of staff from the multi-disciplinary team. It also gives staff easier access to information on the patient and their family's physical, social and emotional well-being and the coping mechanisms they adopt while being treated in either setting.

Some of the management of a child's treatment can often be carried out at the local 'shared care' hospital, where the amount of inpatient and outpatient care is undertaken according to the facilities available. It is obviously more difficult to provide specialist paediatric oncology care on a general paediatric ward but good communication, liaison and education from regional centres to shared care hospitals allows children to receive care much nearer to their home.

Some centres have a satellite pharmacy and haematology laboratory service within their unit; this arrangement considerably reduces the length of time families spend in hospital. Special arrangements with departments such as the haematology laboratories, transfusion department and pharmacy can also reduce outpatient waiting time, providing a smoother hospital visit.

Patient and family education

It is an essential part of ambulatory care that continued education and the reinforcement of practical skills taught as an inpatient are available to both patients and their families. It should never be assumed that information that has been given to families, particularly during their first admission at diagnosis, has been absorbed and, more importantly, understood. It has been shown in many studies that only a small percentage of information is retained during a consultation, and improvements in patient and family education are important (Fredette, 1990).

There has been a great shift towards and gradual acceptance by health care professionals, especially nursing staff, of undertaking a role more as an educator and supporter rather than solely a provider of practical care and procedures that can easily be performed by the family (Popper, 1990). This can only occur if the family are willing and competent to undertake various practical skills and if they are given the correct teaching, guidance and support needed to provide this safely and effectively for their child, thus establishing a partnership in care between health care professionals and families (Casey, 1993). Skills and information taught to families during a hospital admission must be followed up during outpatient visits. Certain procedures that can be carried out at home by the parents or older children themselves can reduce inpatient, outpatient and community health care professionals' time and workload. More importantly, it can allow the family to feel that they have some control and active participation in their child's treatment. Areas include:

- being aware of signs and symptoms of infection, able to monitor the situation through informed teaching and accurate temperature-taking, and management of this situation should it occur
- caring for the child's central venous line by changing dressings and observing the exit site for signs of infection, such as redness, oozing or swelling
- maintaining patency of central venous line by flushing intravenously on a regular basis according to hospital policy
- the administration of intravenous antibiotics through a central venous line
- the administration of bolus intravenous cytotoxic drugs, subcutaneous injections and oral medication.

Documentation

Traditionally, in ambulatory care settings, little documentation of nursing intervention has been undertaken. This reflects, perhaps, the low status of outpatient services, the nature of the work that nurses in these areas have traditionally undertaken and the lack of understanding of the nursing care needs of the patient groups. Inadequate written evidence of clinical decision-making and care provision can put patients at risk (UKCC, 1993). Documentation is required to meet the disparate but interdependent demands of high-quality ambulatory care.

An ambulatory care unit provides complex care involving both therapeutic and organisational issues; there is the capacity to evolve vast amounts of paperwork in an effort to meet both service management and patient care needs. The high patient–nurse ratio and the rapid daily turnover of patients leaves nurses little time for record-keeping. Documentation therefore needs to be easy to use and provide worthwhile, accessible information of practical benefit if it is to be valued. It is necessary to minimise duplication of effort and ensure that information is readily available while maintaining patient confidentiality. Several styles of documentation have been devised: narrative records, charts and flow sheets, dictated records and care plans have all been described (Behrend, 1994).

Patient care issues

Documents are required that provide for each patient a record not only of drugs administered, but also of the nursing care given in relation to the safe administration of chemotherapy and the management of side-effects (Bru *et al.*, 1985; Pickett, 1992).

Pre-printed 'core' care plans that outline specific chemotherapy protocols, management of treatment-related side-effects and investigative procedures have been developed in some centres. This can reduce time spent on paperwork, particularly if the records are designed to be 're-used' (updated) for a patient's consecutive admissions. Such documents can give structure for care-planning by recording assessment (physical and psycho-social), negotiated family participation in care, nursing interventions and evaluation.

Patient records that avoid jargon and clearly explain treatments, the potential side-effects and their management, can play a valuable role in family education, making it intrinsic to planning nursing care. This is especially important in ambulatory nursing care, as each family must be equipped with the information and skills to care for their child at home following treatment. However, the limited time that families spend in the unit reduces the opportunities for such education to take place.

By developing individualised, continuing records of each patient's treatment, their family's nursing needs, the care given and its outcomes, an ongoing document is achieved that promotes continuity of care over time (potentially many years) and between professionals.

The development of parent-held records in some centres (Hully and Hine, 1993; Hooker and Williams, 1996) represents nurses' efforts to meet the needs of families and professionals for information throughout the duration of treatment and beyond, and the desire to enhance care delivery across provider boundaries.

Organisational issues

Much of the success, or otherwise, of a day care admission relies on the planning undertaken by nursing staff. With regard to managing the unit, documentation is required that facilitates pre-admission planning, for example investigations or treatments, the involvement of other disciplines, shared care and community services. Computerised patient administration systems have been adapted with some success to plan the often complex requirements of children attending the ambulatory oncology unit and to allow support services, for example haematology, radiology and pharmacy, to plan for the fluctuating daily workload. This also enables families to be given appointments that more realistically reflect the service they can expect by co-ordinating the input of the various disciplines.

Patient dependency and nursing workload data relevant to ambulatory care are required in order to determine appropriate nursing numbers and skill mix. Existing oncology inpatient classification systems are inappropriate for ambulatory care, as they cannot reflect the complexity of the setting and the multiple variables that influence nursing workload (Medvec, 1994). The realistic documentation of nursing activity is therefore necessary for quality assurance, including the audit of Patient's (Department of Health, 1992) and Children's Charter (Department of Health, 1996) standards and other local and national policies, and to ensure the provision of effective, efficient services.

Professional issues

To promote excellence in professional nursing practice, adequate record-keeping is required to provide a legal document of care and to clarify accountability. This is a particular issue in ambulatory care, where the expansion of nursing roles and responsibilities has blurred the professional boundaries between nurses and other disciplines. To enhance staff development, nursing records can support clinical supervision by providing a focus for discussion and problem-solving by individuals and within groups, for example using critical incident analysis.

Meaningful documentation enables the development of clinical guidelines, protocols and standards of care. Research activities and practice development initiatives are also supported.

Developing nursing practice

The nursing role in oncology ambulatory care has traditionally been largely confined to the administrative and house-keeping aspects of ensuring that clinics run smoothly and of providing practical assistance to medical staff (Tighe *et al.*, 1985). There is an increased need for teams of well-qualified nurses to develop services and provide care that meet the needs of both child and family throughout their cancer experience. Current professional issues within the field include exploring the role of the nurse within the multidisciplinary team, the expansion of the scope of nursing practice and the development of 'named nurse' initiatives.

Clinical practice

Nursing practice boundaries are expanding as nurses extend their technical skills beyond the administration of chemotherapy to include venepuncture, cannulation, the administration of radioactive isotopes and peripheral stem cell harvesting. Formalised nurse practitioner roles that include undertaking bone marrow aspiration and lumbar puncture are being initiated, along with nurse prescribing according to protocol. In addition to the acquisition of technical skills, nurses are also seeking greater responsibility for assessment and clinical decision-making, with regard to administering chemotherapy, advice and family education, making direct referrals to other disciplines, planning the location and timing of therapy and managing supportive care related to side-effects.

Co-ordinating the multidisciplinary team

It is common practice for ambulatory care nursing staff to co-ordinate all the treatment received outside the inpatient ward. This includes care given in the unit itself, in the home by both parents and community nurses and in local hospitals (shared care hospitals). In order to meet the needs of patients and their families, the ambulatory care nurse must be able to co-ordinate the input of many disciplines (Figure 7.1). The development of effective communication networks is therefore vital in ambulatory care, in which the numerous professionals and multiple locations involved may easily result in care becoming fragmented.

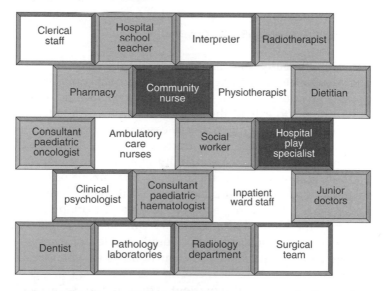

Figure 7.1 The multidisciplinary team – communication and co-ordination are vital

As each admission is of comparatively short duration (usually 1–8 hours), the efforts of these multiple professionals must be managed effectively during this time for maximum patient and family benefit. Nurse-led multidisciplinary meetings can be held that enable nurses to co-ordinate and support the input of individual team members according to the needs of each family and to make appropriate referrals to other members or seek their professional advice.

Primary nursing

The implementation of primary nursing offers great potential for developing nursing roles and service provision within ambulatory care. The long-term nature of the association between families and the oncology centre makes the setting and the speciality eminently suited to primary nursing, offering the potential to improve the continuity of care (Paradise and Kendall, 1985).

Named nurse initiatives give each nurse within a team responsibility for managing a patient caseload, with whom they develop an ongoing relationship, and families have consistent contact with a specific member of the ambulatory care team.

Service development

Nurses in ambulatory care are continually involved in assessing whether treatments currently given as an inpatient could be given as a day case, whether the use of 'home from home' facilities overnight could be utilised to extend the range of complex care offered, and whether treatments now given as day cases could be given at home, by either parents or community nurses. It is vital that nurses are instrumental in assessing the suitability of a new treatment for day case administration and that the nursing assessment of each individual family, including their preferences, is taken into account. Such changes have an obvious impact on facilities and working practices.

Extending the hours that ambulatory care facilities open, either into the evening or at weekends, would enable day care staff to offer more choice to patients and their families of when treatment is delivered.

To ensure that high-quality patient care continues to be available during such service expansions, nursing staff numbers and profiles must reflect increasing patient numbers and patient dependency, as 'sicker' children attend day care for increasingly complex treatments, and reflect expanding practice boundaries, as nurses take on roles previously regarded as medical. Current concerns are that such role developments, initially nurse led, are at risk of being defined by business managers in an attempt to maximise cost-effectiveness. It is imperative that expanding roles are incorporated within nursing care, rather than technical skills being applied in a task-orientated fashion under the direction of medical staff.

Conclusion

Paediatric oncology ambulatory care is an ever-growing and developing area, ranging from pre-diagnosis investigations to cure and long-term follow-up, or palliative and bereavement care. Regional paediatric oncology centres allow for the development of expertise and specialist care both in the inpatient and outpatient settings, and close liaison between these two areas is very important.

Advances in treatment methods and protocols have enabled more day care treatment to take place. It is therefore essential that an increase in education of families and shared care hospitals takes place, so that a partnership develops towards the full management of the child with cancer from all carers involved.

Documentation of nursing care is of extreme importance from a practical, organisational and legal aspect. It should form a concise but integral part of patient care to enable safe practice and efficient communication between members of the multidisciplinary team.

Development of nurses' extended clinical roles and responsibilities should be reflected through appropriate training, the recognition of additional workload and responsibilities held and adequate staffing levels and facilities to mirror this.

The future of paediatric oncology ambulatory care is assured – nurses in this field are ideally placed to be both proactive and creative in designing services that can best meet the needs of children and families.

References

Behrend, S.W. (1994) Documentation in the ambulatory setting. *Seminars in Oncology Nursing*, **10**(4): 264–80.

Brenner, A. (1994) Caring for children during procedure: a review of the literature. *Pediatric Nursing*, **20**(5): 451–8.

Broome, M.E. (1994) Children's medical fears, coping behaviour patterns and pain perceptions during a lumbar puncture. *European Journal of Cancer Care*, **3**: 31–8.

Bru, G.A., Viamontes, C.M., Nirenberg, A. and Poremba, F.A. (1985) Short form for short stay. *American Journal of Nursing*, **85**(4): 401–3.

Casey, A. (1993) Development and use of the partnership model of nursing care, in Glasper, E.A. and Tucker, A. (eds) *Advances in Child Health Nursing*. (London: Scutari Press).

Department of Health (1992) *The Patient's Charter*. (HMSO: London).

Department of Health (1996) *The Patient's Charter – Services for Children and Young People*. (HMSO: London).

Eiser, C. and Havermans, T. (1994) Long term social adjustment after treatment for childhood cancer. *Archives of Disease in Childhood*, **70**(1): 66–70.

Fredette, S.L. (1990) A model for improving cancer patient education. *Cancer Nursing*, **13**(4): 207–15.

Hooker, L. and Williams, J. (1996) Parent-held shared care records: bridging the communication gaps. *British Journal of Nursing*, **5**(12): 738–41.

Hully, M. and Hine, J. (1993) Using parent-held records in an oncology unit. *Paediatric Nursing*, **5**(8): 14–16.

Kissen, G.D.N. and Wallace, W.H.B. (1995) *Long Term Follow Up Therapy Based Guidelines*. (Leicester: The United Kingdom's Children's Cancer Study Group Late Effects Group).

Medvec, B.R. (1994) Productivity and workload measurement in ambulatory oncology. *Seminars in Oncology Nursing*, **10**(4): 288–95.

Nail, L.M., Green, D., Jones, L.S. and Flannery, M. (1989) Nursing care by telephone: describing practice in an ambulatory oncology centre. *Oncology Nursing Forum*, **16**(3): 387–95.

NHS Management Executive (1993) *Day Surgery. Training and Education. Section 5*. Report from the Day Surgery Task Force. (London: HMSO).

Paradise, R.L. and Kendall, V.M. (1985) Ambulatory care: primary nursing brings continuity. *Nursing Management*, **16**(12): 27–30.

Pickett, R.R. (1992) Outpatient oncology chemotherapy documentation tool. *Oncology Nursing Forum*, **19**(3): 515–17.

Popper, B. (1990) A parent's perspective: the changing role of parents' involvement in the health care system. *Children's Health Care*, **19**: 242–3.

Reams, C.A. (1990) Inpatients and outpatients on one unit. *Journal of Paediatric Nursing*, **7**(2): 77–8.

Tighe, M.G., Fisher, S.G., Hastings, C. and Heller, D. (1985) A study of the oncology nurse role in ambulatory care. *Oncology Nursing Forum*, **12**(6): 23-7.

UKCC (1993) *Standards for Records and Record Keeping*. (London: UKCC).

8

THE ROLE OF THE MACMILLAN PAEDIATRIC NURSING SERVICE

Margaret Evans and Anne Thompson

Key points

- Due to improved survival rates in childhood cancer, there is now a greater emphasis on psychosocial issues and early discharge.
- Macmillan paediatric nursing teams have developed in response to the need for a multidisciplinary support structure for families.
- Research has shown that palliative care for children with cancer should be provided in the home setting, and Macmillan nurses have the expertise to promote this.
- Macmillan nurses need to ensure that they fulfil the role of the specialist nurse and that this is recognised.

Introduction

This chapter will look at how the Macmillan paediatric nurse has developed in the ambulatory care setting and in the context of paediatric oncology. The role of the clinical nurse specialist will be discussed, as this is an important issue in relation to such posts, particularly in the present economic climate. It will then explain how the nurse functions as a clinical specialist, demonstrating how this role forms an integral part of the ambulatory care philosophy.

Developments in the field of paediatric oncology have resulted in a greater emphasis on psychosocial care for for the child with cancer, and on early discharge into the community. Macmillan paediatric nursing teams have therefore been set up in regional centres to promote this philosophy and are very much a part of the ambulatory care setting.

The success of this approach is largely dependent upon an appropriate multidisciplinary support structure to reflect the family's individual needs and circumstances, one which will ensure 24-hour access to appropriate and knowlegeable advice and care, especially during the palliative stages of the child's illness.

It is important, therefore, that Macmillan nurses fulfil the role of a clinical nurse specialist to promote high standards of care and to co-ordinate a complex support structure effectively.

Childhood cancer

Childhood cancer is rare, affecting 1 in 600 children in the UK (Kohler, 1991). Thirty years ago, this disease was considered to be acute and terminal, but today, with a cure rate of at least 60 per cent across the range of childhood cancers, it is considered to be a chronic life-threatening illness (Birch, 1988). This still means, however, that it is responsible for over 400 deaths per year (Goldman *et al.*, 1990).

The improvement in prognosis has largely been due to the development of controlled clinical trials using combination chemotherapy, and to the centralisation of treatment (Stiller, 1994). All 22 regional paediatric oncology centres in the UK carry out increasingly intensive and complex treatment, under the guidance of the United Kingdom Children's Cancer Study Group and the Medical Research Council. This co-operative strategy has proved to be the most effective way of evaluating new treatment protocols when numbers of patients are small. Improvements in survival have had far-reaching implications in terms of psychosocial support for families, and it is only relatively recently that regional centres have placed strong emphasis on the importance of educating and ongoing support.

Faulkner *et al.* (1993) have suggested that the uncertainty of survival poses problems that can be as challenging as facing death, and Martinson *et al.* (1990) have emphasised the fact that the extended period of uncertainty affects the lives of all the family members. Koocher and O'Malley (1981) have studied the psychosocial consequences of surviving childhood cancer. They believe that survivors are at risk of emotional disturbance and should receive interventions designed to reduce social isolation and provide family support. Norman and Bennett (1986) reinforced this in a study that found that the greatest amount of the community nurse's time (67 per cent) was spent in the provision of emotional support for the child and family.

Home care

The recommendation that early discharge to home care for all hospitalised children should be instituted, if at all possible, has been well documented over the years. Home care undoubtedly encourages a return to normality and a subsequent improvement in quality of life for the child and family, and professionals have identified the obvious benefits of this for the child with cancer (Patel, 1990; Evans and Kelly, 1995).

Effective community nursing support allows the family to remain intact for as much of the time as possible, and they are able to make an earlier and quicker adjustment to a long-term illness. In addition and more importantly, parents feel more in control because they are enabled to manage their child's care. This also seems to be true when parents care for their child at home during terminal illness.

Various studies on home care for children dying of cancer have suggested that not only do the children themselves feel happier at home, but also their parents cope better with bereavement if they have been able to care for their child at home during a terminal illness.

Martinson *et al.* (1978) were the first to document a study looking at home care for dying children. The aim was to examine the feasibility and desirability of the home as an alternative to the hospital for children whose death from cancer was impending. Their findings indicated that, in order for home care to be successful, the child, the parents and the physician needed to perceive the service as a viable alternative and that the nurses supporting the parents needed to be experienced in home care. Parents valued the service because they could be involved in care and the family could be reunited. The children were able to die in familiar and more natural surroundings.

Kohler and Radford (1985) interviewed the parents of 18 children who had died from cancer. They found that all but one family had decided to look after their child at home, but that their anxieties would have been eased had they been given more information and support.

Goldman *et al.* (1990) reviewed the setting for palliative care – home, hospital or hospice. They argued that home will always be the place of preference for the child but that the family need to feel comfortable with this choice. Hospital, although familiar, has obvious disadvantages, and most families find it inappropriate to adapt to new surroundings and new faces in the hospice setting. They made the important point that, with appropriate expertise and support, it is possible to provide palliative care to children in their own homes.

The specialist role of the Macmillan paediatric nurse

This role has evolved in response to the need for ongoing support at home, throughout the course of the child's treatment and during palliative care should that become necessary. Unlike their adult care counterparts, Macmillan paediatric nurses care for children across the illness trajectory (Table 8.1), and because their case load is small and care more intensive, they travel much greater distances. By 'outreaching' from the regional paediatric oncology centre, the nurses are able to provide a vital link with the community and enhance ambulatory care.

Initially, most of the posts were set up using a community nursing model similar to that described by Lessing and Tatman (1991), in which direct hands-on care was provided and although the nurses were hospital based, they were not necessarily seen as clinical nurse specialists.

Today, perhaps because the role of the clinical nurse specialist is more clearly defined, Macmillan paediatric nurses are expected to fulfil that role (Webber, 1994) and have become recognised as highly skilled and knowledgeable in their field.

Castledine (1995) has emphasised the need for clarity, particularly in the light of the specialist proposals outlined in the final PREP report (UKCC, 1997). Webber (1994) has identified four key components of the role of the clinical nurse specialist – teaching, research, leadership and clinical expertise. She has highlighted the fact that the Macmillan nurse can promote high standards of care by acting as a catalyst and an agent of change (Table 8.2).

Wilson-Barnett (1995) suggests that specialist nurses should be aiming to make themselves redundant by their role as co-ordinators and educators of other members of the primary health care team. It is certainly true that, for Macmillan paediatric services, the balance of direct and indirect care is changing, as more generic paediatric community nursing teams are being set up.

Table 8.1 Aspects of specific support and care at key times of the disease trajectory

Diagnosis	Ensuring that children and their families understand appropriately the implications of the disease and its treatment
	Giving confidence to parents to meet the physical and psychological needs of their child
	Co-ordinating an integral approach to care
When treatment regimens completed	Recognising that the atmosphere of celebration is tempered by insecurities, anxieties and continuing uncertainty
	Affording opportunities to discuss fears of relapse or possible long-term effects of treatment.
	Encouraging the family to complete their return to 'normal' life
At relapse	Helping families to come to terms with the implications of recurrent disease
When cure is no longer possible	Offering counselling and support, so that families can make important decisions and choices
	Providing specialist knowledge and skills to enable complex palliative care to be managed at home when desired
	Enabling families to retain control over care and ownership of their child's death
Throughout all stages of the disease trajectory	Providing information/education/skill training in order to increase feelings of confidence and independence, and the child's and family's ability to retain control
	Co-ordinating an integrated multidisciplinary approach to care by liaising between primary, secondary or tertiary sectors
	Bridging gaps in care by being available to complement and extend existing service where appropriate
	Ensuring that school personnel have access to adequate information and community to enable them to meet their own as well as the child's needs

Table 8.2 Components of the multidimensional role of the Macmillan paediatric nurse as a clinical nurse specialist

Clinical expertise	Teaching	Leadership	Research
Empowerment	Reflect current knowledge and practice	Role model	Analyse
Partnership	Innovate	Resource	Utilise
Advocate	Stimulate	Co-ordinator	Disseminate
Specialist knowledge and skills	Multidisciplinary	Advisor	Assist
Direct care giver	Clinical placements	Change agent	Initiate
		Indirect care	

This makes it all the more important clearly to identify the specific role of the Macmillan paediatric nurse. Bignold *et al.* (1994) have commented that, for parents, the fact that professionals 'have been there before' matters most of all to them. Based on their research, they find it impossible to see how parents' individual needs could be met by more generic services that are not a part of the specialist framework of care and are therefore seen as outside the 'culture' of childhood cancer.

The culture of childhood cancer

Bignold *et al.* (1994) found that families frequently differentiate between specialist and non-specialist care. Families recognise and value the expertise and honest open approach of the specialist health professionals, often viewing themselves and the specialist team as being 'insiders' to the culture and 'community' of childhood cancer. In contrast, general practitioners and other members of the primary health care team will possibly see one or two children with cancer during their entire career. They are therefore disadvantaged by the lack of opportunity to gain experience, which leads many to express concerns regarding their ability to offer appropriate support.

Families who perceive a lack of specific expertise or a different approach may think of the primary health care team or local hospital as 'outside' the culture of childhood cancer. Unfortunately, this can undermine the family's confidence and result in a reluctance to accept 'outside' support, which, unless addressed, can produce gaps in care provision.

As an 'insider', the Macmillan paediatric nurse can play a vital role in counteracting this perception. Creating collaborative relationships with the primary health care team and local hospital, and acting as an adviser and resource, promotes opportunities to share care, thus drawing the generalist team into the multidisciplinary support structure (Figure 8.1).

Collaboration with the multidisciplinary team

Although recognising that most families prefer early discharge to home-based care whenever possible, it is nevertheless important to acknowledge that parents will continue to have anxieties and fears.

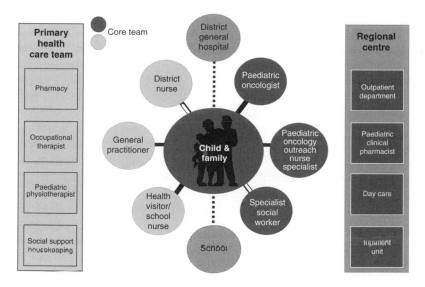

Figure 8.1

Many families express concerns that they may feel isolated and unsupported, and lack confidence at home. Equally, families often fear being swamped by professionals. By addressing these issues, reassurance can be given to the families that they will not be abandoned, that they will be helped to retain control over their situation and that a support structure will be developed with the aim of reflecting their individual needs, circumstances and wishes. Most importantly, particularly in the palliative and terminal stages of the child's illness, the family will want to know that they have round-the-clock access to an effective support team, able to offer appropriate and knowledgeable advice and care (Figure 8.1). Appointing a key co-ordinator and family advocate is therefore crucial. The Macmillan paediatric nurse is often identified as the most appropriate person to undertake this role, and the success of this approach is clearly demonstrated at many major treatment centres.

Palliative care

As previously stated, the child's home is almost always the place of choice for palliative care. However, without the availability of considerable support, many children would die in hospital. The support that families receive while caring for a dying child has many consequences. It will influence the decisions and choices that the family make, the quality of the child's remaining life, how the family cope with the dying process, their lasting memories and the way in which they are able to work through their grief while learning to live with the death of their child. Facilitating optimal support during the palliative stage of a child's illness is, therefore, given the highest priority by Macmillan paediatric nurses. The effective use of interpersonal skills in order to cross professional boundaries will ensure that families do not experience gaps in care at this vital time.

How their child might die and the fear of pain or uncontrollable symptoms are often the greatest concerns expressed by parents. Ensuring that the family and members of the multidisciplinary team are prepared in advance for the onset and management of symptoms, and eventually the death of the child, will minimise the risk of panic situations and helps the family to maintain a sense of control. By developing specialist knowledge, expertise and skills, particularly in the area of symptom management and palliative care, the nurse is able to complement existing services, enabling children requiring even intense and complex care to be supported at home until their death (Figure 8.2).

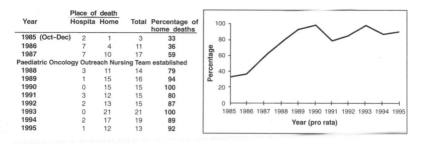

Year	Place of death		Total	Percentage of home deaths
	Hospital	Home		
1985 (Oct–Dec)	2	1	3	33
1986	7	4	11	36
1987	7	10	17	59
Paediatric Oncology Outreach Nursing Team established				
1988	3	11	14	79
1989	1	15	16	94
1990	0	15	15	100
1991	3	12	15	80
1992	2	13	15	87
1993	0	21	21	100
1994	2	17	19	89
1995	1	12	13	92

Figure 8.2

Again, by promoting an empowerment and partnership approach, it is hoped that individual family members will be able to live with the death of their child, comfortable with their own role and the role of others, thus minimising feelings of guilt, anger and regret.

Macmillan paediatric nurses continue to offer support during the initial bereavement phase but need to identify an appropriate time to 'safely' withdraw from the family, while ensuring that continuing support is available from other agencies. They must also take care to address their own emotional needs. Having been involved with families for often considerable lengths of time, their feelings of loss should not be underestimated.

Many Macmillan paediatric nurses are developing the use of reflective practice, clinical supervision and personal counselling as a means of obtaining ongoing support.

Education

The role of the Macmillan paediatric nurse is relatively new. Modelling good practice and raising awareness of the role has produced a demand to contribute to a wide range of educational opportunities across many disciplines and settings.

Of particular importance are areas where there is a lack of experience in the care of children with cancer and their families – the community, local hospitals and schools. Increasing the level of knowledge and skills encourages involvement and promotes appropriate care.

In addition, the majority of children with progressive disease are now being cared for at home and die at home, and there is an increasing recognition that inpatient nursing and medical personnel are becoming deskilled in the management of children at this stage of their disease. This loss of skills and expertise, particularly in relation to symptom management, also has implications for the care of children at other stages of the disease trajectory (see Table 8.1).

Many Macmillan paediatric nurses are now attempting to address these issues through education and through acting as a clinical resource. Again, it is important that their role is recognised as that of a specialist nurse and that they have the background and vision to fulfil that role.

Conclusion

An audit carried out at Southampton found that the provision of information and support forms the basis of the role of the Macmillan paediatric nurse. This was clearly the aspect of their role which parents valued most highly, and a questionnaire that followed the audit supported this (Evans and Kelly, 1995). Although this work provided a means of data collection, the findings were largely qualitative in nature, and it is still necessary to find a more precise quantitative methodology to audit standards of care based on measurable data.

In the USA, Martinson et al. (1978) and Lauer and Camitta (1980) were able to demonstrate through their research that community services for children with cancer were cost-effective, and it is clear that Macmillan services will be required to do likewise.

Webber (1994) has commented that the review and reform of the NHS is exerting a major influence on Macmillan nursing services in that they are required to demonstrate their value to purchasers of health care – not only in terms of providing a quality service, but also in terms of cost-effectiveness.

Notter has made an important point in relation to the future of specialist nurses, and this applies, of course, to Macmillan paediatric nurses:

> Specialist nurses need to find a way of describing their practice that leaves managers and purchasers in no doubt about the level of service they offer and the contribution they make to the provision of high-quality care. (Notter, 1995, p. 1330)

At the same time, looking at purely measurable factors is not enough. Bignold *et al.* (1994) have made the point that it is tempting for health care planners to compare care in specialist and generalist hospitals by using easily measurable factors such as cost-effectiveness or travelling time.

These factors do, of course, matter, but their data show that 'climate' and cultural factors are, in the view of parents, fundamental to their experience of good-quality care.

The market philosophy that has now become an integral part of the NHS places an increasingly strong emphasis on quantity rather than quality, and it is for this reason that standards of care could be compromised. The onus is, therefore, on Macmillan paediatric nurses, as part of the ambulatory care setting, to ensure that quality issues are given priority in the service they provide to children and their families.

Table 8.3 Macmillan paediatric nurse in collaboration with the child and family

Goal	Intervention
Open trusting relationship	Explain the role of the Macmillan paediataric nurse
	Establish confidence in service by discussing expertise, continuity and responsiveness
	Non-judgemental, befriending approach
	Provide positive reinforcement, openness and active involvement
	Enable child/parent to express feelings, concerns and stressors
Partnership	Develop a collaborative partnership approach
	Jointly formulate care plan to reflect child's/family's personalities, preferences and coping strategies
Empowerment	Affirm parents' role as primary care givers
	Reinforce parents' ability to provide expert care
	Increase confidence and ability to retain control by providing information, education and skill training
Advocacy	Support child's and parents' rights to receive holistic and individualised care, shaped by their own decisions and choices

References

Bignold, S., Ball, S. and Crib, A. (1994) *Nursing Families of Children with Cancer: A Research Summary*. (London: Cancer Relief MacMillan Fund).

Birch, J.M. (1988) Improvements in survivors in childhood cancer: results of a population based survey over 30 years. *British Medical Journal*, **296**: 1372–6.

Castledine, G. (1995) Editorial: Defining specialist nursing. *British Journal of Nursing*, **4**(5): 264–5.

Evans, M. and Kelly, P. (1995) Bringing support home for families of children with cancer. *British Journal of Nursing*, **4**(7): 395–401.

Faulkner, A., Peace, G. and O'Keefe, C. (1993) Future imperfect. *Nursing Times*, **89**(51): 40–2.

Goldman, A., Beardsmore, S. and Hunt, J. (1990) Palliative care for children with cancer – home, hospital or hospice. *Archives of Diseases in Childhood*, **65**(6): 641–3.

Kohler, J. (1991) Recent advances in the management of paediatric cancer. *Postgraduate Update*, **42**(10): 950–60.

Kohler, J.A. and Radford, M. (1985) Terminal care for children dying of cancer: quantity and quality of life. *British Medical Journal*, **291**: 115–16.

Koocher, G.E. and O'Malley, J.E. (1981) *The Damocles Syndrome. Psychosocial Consequences of Surviving Childhood Cancer*. (New York: McGraw-Hill).

Lauer, M.E. and Camitta, B.M. (1980) Home care for dying children: a nursing model. *Journal of Paediatrics*, **97**(6): 1032–5.

Lessing, D. and Tatman, M.A. (1991) Paediatric home care in the 1990s. *Archives of Diseases in Childhood*, **66**(8): 994–6.

Martinson, I.M., Armstrong, G.D., Geis, D.P. *et al.* (1978) Home care for children dying of cancer. *Pediatrics*, **62**(1): 106–13.

Martinson, I.M., Gilliss, C., Coughlin Colaizzo, D., Freeman, M. and Bossert, E. (1990) Impact of childhood cancer on healthy school-age siblings. *Cancer Nursing*, **13**(3): 183–90.

Norman, R. and Bennett, M. (1986) Care of the dying child at home: a unique co-operative relationship. *Australian Journal of Advanced Nursing*, **3**(4): 3–16.

Notter, J. (1995) Marketing specialist practice to managers and purchasers. *British Journal of Nursing*, **4**(22): 1330–4.

Patel, N. (1990) The child with cancer in the community, in Thompson, J. (ed.) *The Child With Cancer*. (London: Scutari Press).

Stiller, C.A. (1994) Centralised treatment, entry to trials and survival. *British Journal of Cancer*, **70**: 352–62.

UKCC (1997) *PREP and You*. (London: UKCC).

Webber, J. (1994) A model response. *Nursing Times*, **90**(25): 66–8.

Wilson-Barnett, J. (1995) Specialism in nursing: effectiveness and maximization of benefit. *Journal of Advanced Nursing*, **1**(21): 1–2.

9

NURSE-LED CLINICS IN AMBULATORY CARE

Yvonne Fulton and Linda Phillips

The nurse-led clinic could perhaps be considered as the logical outcome of the expanded role of the nurse within ambulatory paediatrics. In this chapter, different models of nurse-led clinic will be outlined, and as an example, the setting up of an enuresis clinic by the second author will be discussed in detail. The advantages for patients, nurses and the health service will be identified, and inherent difficulties will be analysed. Finally, the implications for the future of nurse-led clinics will be evaluated.

In the context of this chapter, a clinic in ambulatory care is defined as a period of time set aside by a health professional to see patients with a particular condition. A nurse-led clinic is one in which the nurse takes responsibility for the consultation with the patient. Within these clinics, guidelines to provide a framework for the work undertaken are usually developed by nurses, managers and medical staff.

The concept of the nurse-led clinic is not a new one, and indeed the earliest descriptions come from within paediatric nursing itself. The paediatric nurse practitioner programmes in the USA during the 1960s prepared nurses with baccalaureate or Master's degrees to undertake an expanded role in providing total health care for children. The impetus for this nursing development was to save physicians' time in areas of inadequate health provision in private practice. It arose in response to changing health care needs and increasing medical costs in the USA and to the perceived inability of doctors to deal with minor health problems. The nurse could provide a cheaper service and deal more effectively with minor problems (Stilwell, 1988). Some of these conditions exist in the UK today and are being reflected in the changing provision of health care.

Although the nurse-led clinic in the hospital setting is just beginning its evolution, there is a long and strong tradition of such clinics within UK primary care. Health visitors have for many years held regular drop-in clinics for mothers with infants and toddlers, providing a range of services such as health and development checks, health education and advice on minor ailments. Recently, there has been further impetus for nurse-led clinics within primary care because of the many changes in general practice. With the inception of the new contract in 1990, general practitioners have had to provide a range of screening and health promotion programmes. The Health of the Nation health reforms have placed more emphasis on preventative health work and increased the drive to boost immunisation rates. Clinical audit has identified a need for more preventative work in chronic conditions such as asthma and diabetes. Thus general practice workload has increased at the same time as general practitioner fundholding has provided an incentive for the introduction of a more economical skill mix within practices.

These factors have provided the impetus for a large increase in the number of nurses employed in general practice (Hampson, 1994). Practice nurses run a range of clinics including childhood immunisation clinics and asthma clinics. Increasingly, health visitors, practice nurses and school nurses hold clinics for young people on aspects of health education such as drugs, sexual health and self-esteem (Millar and Booth, 1996). Family psychosocial support, for example positive parenting programmes for parents in vulnerable families (Angeli *et al.*, 1994), is also given.

There is also a growing trend for practice nurses to treat children for minor ailments, for example during the sessions described by Rees and Kinnersley (1996). In the UK, the 'paediatric nurse practitioner' role is being undertaken within A&E departments (Kobryn and Pearce, 1991). These nurses diagnose and prescribe care and preventative treatment for a wide range of minor injuries. They are also able to prescribe, although this power is currently extremely limited.

As can be seen, the nurse-led clinic is well established within community settings and is developing to keep pace with changing health needs. Many of these clinics are led by nurses who are practising at the level of advanced nursing. The UKCC (1994) describes advanced nursing practice as pioneering new roles in response to changing health care needs. However, in reality, the nurses leading the clinics have varying levels of autonomy, which depend on local factors. Such factors will include the skill, confidence and aspirations of the nurse, the vision and innovation promoted by managers and the level of power-sharing the medical staff are willing to accept.

Within ambulatory paediatric nursing, such clinics have been slower to emerge but are now evolving in several different ways. These innovations are closely linked with the development of advanced nursing practice, which can be divided into two categories: the clinical nurse specialist and the nurse practitioner (Read and Graves, 1994). A comparison of the definitions of these two concepts will inform the discussion at this point.

The International Council of Nurses (1992) proposes that:

> the nurse specialist is a nurse prepared beyond the level of a nurse generalist and authorised to practise as a specialist with advanced expertise in a branch of the nursing field. Speciality practice includes clinical, teaching, administration, research and consultant roles.

Barbara Stilwell pioneered the role of the nurse practitioner in the UK. Stilwell *et al.* (1987) define the role thus:

> The Nurse Practitioner in primary care settings practises an advanced, expanded nursing role and makes professionally autonomous decisions, taking sole responsibility. She/he receives clients with undifferentiated, undiagnosed problems. She/he diagnoses, prescribes and provides care, works closely with other professionals and respects professional boundaries.

The paediatric nurse-led clinics which exist in the UK today within the hospital setting receive children with a particular problem already diagnosed. In this, they differ from nurse practitioner clinics in the USA and in UK general practice where patients can present with problems that require initial diagnosis.

Currently then, within the hospital setting, nurse-led clinics are an extension of the role of the clinical nurse specialist. These clinics are often developed as a result of a recognised need by the nursing team and consultant in a particular speciality, such as diabetes, asthma or cystic fibrosis, for patients to receive more teaching and counselling than can be given at a consultant's clinic. The daily management of such conditions requires detailed ongoing support and advice, which some consultants appreciate that they do not have the time to give.

Such clinics are on a continuum of different levels of consultant involvement. At one end of the continuum, clinics have joint appointments with medical staff and shared decision-making between nurse and doctor (Palmer, 1995). At the other end, nurses are running clinics independently of medical staff. An example of the latter is the diabetes clinic at Southampton held fortnightly by the diabetes nurse specialist. Children and their families are invited to drop in to see the nurse for advice, to see a range of equipment and to pick up information. The nurse will adjust insulin doses if necessary, and there is no medical involvement.

Another example of a clinic with high levels of nurse autonomy is to be found within the open referral asthma clinic in Brighton (Wooler, 1993). The respiratory nurses who run this clinic take referrals from general practitioners, health visitors and practice nurses in the area on a 'please see and advise' basis. The nurses are able to prescribe inhaled medication and short-course steroids from a nurses' formulary and to make consultant referrals. However, if a chest X-ray is needed, a medical registrar's signature is required. It could be argued that these are bureaucratic limitations on the nurse's autonomy. If a nurse can make a competent decision on whether a child needs medication, it seems rational to assume that such a nurse will be able to make a competent decision on whether a child needs an X-ray. Read and Graves (1994) recommend that the Department of Health clarify these policy issues.

Having considered nurse-led clinics in general, the next step is to illustrate these issues further by considering the enuresis clinic developed and led by the second author. This initiative took place within an NDU, the children's outpatients department at Southampton University NHS Trust. NDUs are centres of collaborative clinical change where nurses work together to achieve their goals and aspirations (Wright, 1992). It is within such innovative environments that opportunities to expand nursing practice can be negotiated and accepted.

In this instance, it was the nurse who identified the need for a nurse-led clinic and negotiated with her medical colleagues for its introduction. There were difficulties encountered during the implementation stage, but the nurse eventually achieved the autonomy necessary to manage her own patients. The clinic has been very successful, demonstrated by a patient satisfaction survey and the outcome of an audit. Many of the children who have successfully achieved dryness had for years been attending enuresis clinics run by doctors; some had had previous inpatient treatment.

In order to put this clinic into context, it is necessary to clarify the term 'enuresis', which is often used indiscriminately to describe 'wet children'. The child with enuresis has no underlying organic disease. He or she is able to pass urine normally but does so in a socially unacceptable fashion. However, a distinction should be made between the passing of urine at night during sleep (nocturnal enuresis) and the involuntary wetting that occurs during the day when the child is awake (diurnal enuresis).

Nocturnal enuresis is the most prevalent of all childhood problems, with estimates of a half to three-quarters of a million children over 7 years of age regularly suffering with bedwetting in Britain at any one time. While nocturnal enuresis at first might be considered a fairly minor complaint, the problem assumes great importance when observed from the child's perspective. Butler (1994) graphically describes the 'perplexity, humiliation, alienation and verbal and physical abuse' suffered by enuretic children, who will go to enormous lengths to avoid discovery. Toilet-training and toilet accidents are the second most cited problem resulting in child abuse (Kempe and Helfer, 1972). This problem clearly has enormous impact on the health and relationship of child and family.

Many parents do not seek treatment because they believe that the child will grow out of it or because they blame themselves. They experience loss of confidence in their parental skills and are made to feel guilty and anxious. Therefore the care of these children is complex and time-consuming, and requires excellent communication skills and family support. The relationship a nurse can build with the family is an essential component of the successful management of this problem. The time required for consultations during an enuresis clinic is an important resource issue.

Having outlined the problem of enuresis, the next step is to consider the children's care at Southampton that led to the nurse intervention. General practitioners referred children with day- and night-time wetting to a variety of consultant paediatricians and surgeons in the children's outpatients department. Most of the children with night-time wetting were found to have no organic cause for the problem. Those with day-time wetting often had a past history of medical problems but, following medical investigation, were considered to be able to overcome their continence problems themselves.

The management strategies of each consultant varied considerably within the limited clinic time allotted for each child. Some children received verbal advice but with no written literature to reinforce the information. Others were treated with medication.

Those with nocturnal enuresis were often given an alarm with no further support. Some were simply discharged from the clinic.

The parent of a child who was to be treated with an enuresis alarm either had to go on a waiting list until an alarm was available or receive a quick demonstration from an outpatient nurse with limited time available. No records were maintained of to whom alarms had been loaned, so many were lost and those waiting for an alarm had to wait for long periods to receive one.

The nurse recognised that not only would these matters have to be resolved, but the ability to develop a supportive and trusting relationship with the child and family would also be a vital ingredient in the successful management of this problem. Such support did not necessarily have to be given by a doctor. Medicine is about treating a disorder, but once any organic reason for the cause of the bedwetting had been eliminated, the management and support of the child and family could be given by an experienced paediatric nurse. Thus a vision of a nurse-led service within the children's outpatients department was evolved.

Intensive knowledge about enuresis was gained by private study, visiting enuresis clinics, attending study days and undertaking the ENB 978 course on the Promotion of Continence and Management of Incontinence. In order to deliver evidence-based child health nursing (Royal College of Nursing, 1995; Callery, 1997), a thorough literature review and consultation with appropriate specialists was undertaken. For example, Bradbury and Meadow (1995) found that combined treatment with Desmopressin and an enuresis alarm was helpful. This research-based treatment underpinned one of the clinical protocols that was developed with the local consultant's approval. Other protocols were developed from guidelines based on clinical research and current practice recommended by Clark *et al.* (1994) and also from the Enuresis Resource and Information Centre (ERIC).

Having developed a strong knowledge base, the nurse was able to argue with clinicians and managers for autonomy to make her own clinical assessment. She wanted to be able to obtain a detailed history of the child's problem and then exercise her professional judgement to base the child's management on his or her individual needs, using the evidence-based protocols with flexibility.

During the implementation of this clinic, several challenges emerged. One involved the clinic's interface with the consultants. Many of the consultants expressed concerns that a nurse would only be able to follow a strict protocol of management and would not be able to create alternative strategies. Others remained unconvinced that the service was necessary. They felt that patients would expect to see a doctor, rather than a nurse, when attending a hospital appointment. Others remained non-committal, clearly waiting to see what would happen. However, those who became involved in the nurse-led clinic management strategy also became interested in the concept.

In September 1994, the service was formally commenced, and within 3 months the nurse was managing 34 children and receiving new referrals weekly. Many of the children were severe wetters with behavioural disorders or came from families with a history of family stress. There are currently 120 children and families being treated, many children having nephrological and urological as well as family problems.

The success of the nurse-led clinic can be measured by the number of referrals received, the measurable amount of continence achieved by the children and the support for the service from medical colleagues. The nurse was motivated to succeed and demonstrated a positive attitude with each patient attending the clinic. She was able to develop a supportive and trusting relationship with the child and family, who were able to contact her any time they had a problem. However, the emphasis at all times was on empowering the children to take charge of their own problem. At no time has the nurse experienced any concern from parents that they are attending a nurse-led service, although all patients are seen by the consultant within 6 months of their first appointment at the enuresis clinic.

Unfortunately, initiatives such as this can be severely hindered by the currents of imbalance of power between doctors and nurses, and the financial constraints on acute services. While medical staff fight to retain their level of services, nursing initiatives can lose support. This clinic was not reflected in the budget between the purchaser and provider so, as it expanded, there was no funding to sustain it. When money had to be saved, the enuresis clinic was at the top of the list of proposed cuts. However, when the clinic came under threat during a funding crisis, the consultants recognised what they were about to lose and fought to retain it. The precedent has been set, and the clinic has been formally recognised. To have successfully introduced a nurse-led service into the children's outpatients department, where doctors had traditionally taken the lead, was exciting and invigorating. It nevertheless required dedication and motivation. It was recognition of the need for the service that made the nurse strive for it despite initial opposition.

Having analysed the development of one nurse-led clinic, it is worth considering some of the advantages of such clinics. For nurses, there is increased role satisfaction in being able to practise autonomously in the delivery of holistic care (Read and Graves, 1994). Patients benefit too. Evans and Griffiths (1994) point out that, often when patients no longer need medical care, some will come to need 'education, rehabilitation and nurturing', which a nurse-led service is well placed to provide. Patients can benefit from the more relaxed atmosphere in the nurse-led clinic compared with the medical clinic. Wooler (1993) believes that the informal atmosphere provided by respiratory nurses who are not focused on ward routines enables better teaching and learning to take place in the clinic setting than in the hospital ward. Butterworth (1991) cites several studies demonstrating patients' satisfaction with nurse-led ambulatory care, particularly in the caring and supportive role.

Following a patient satisfaction survey on the nurse-led enuresis service, it became apparent that parents found the service better than that provided by doctors. The patients said that nurses were more approachable and knowledgeable. They felt less intimidated and were able to ask questions that received simple explanations.

There are arguments that nurse-led clinics have the potential to save health care resources. A key motivation is the imperative to reduce junior doctors' hours (NHS Management Executive, 1991). In response to this, the Trent region set up and evaluated a project involving 32 expanded nursing roles (Read and Graves, 1994). These roles included nurse-led clinics (although none were within paediatrics) and a neonatal nurse practitioner. The project report concluded that, although these roles had not yet had a major impact on the actual hours that doctors worked, they had affected junior doctors' workload. This was demonstrated by the increased job satisfaction and reduced work intensity of junior doctors.

Other financial implications are demonstrated, for example within the field of asthma care. Madge (1995) found that structured nurse-led discharge planning, including attendance at a nurse-led clinic, reduced readmission rates and reduced morbidity. Wooler (1993) has argued that the provision of a nurse-led asthma clinic may be cost-effective by enhancing treatment and reducing hospital admissions.

Another important advantage is that nurse-led clinics can provide families with much-needed integration between primary and specialist care, as recommended by Thornes (1993). There are, however, several key problems that present themselves when nurses take on the wider scope of practice involved in nurse-led clinics. Clear clinical judgements must be made because the nurse's actions will be judged against those of a reasonable physician (Castledine, 1993). This requires education, experience and the exercise of accountability. Clear employer and professional guidelines are needed, incorporating evidence-based medicine, and nurses developing these roles in the future will need to be educated to Master's level.

Another problem is the concern voiced by some nurses that these nursing roles evolve only under the aegis of medical domination as a cost-cutting exercise or to save medical time. Nurses avow that they do not want to be mini-doctors but wish to be better nurses. However, it could be argued that nurses should not refuse expanded practice because of this. These roles present opportunities to gain experience and satisfaction in working more independently. Undertaking and evaluating such roles gives the opportunity to bring about change in the differential between doctors and nurses. If nurses refuse the expanded role, change will be slow if at all.

Although there are arguments that nurse-led clinics can be cost-effective, there are methodological difficulties in measuring the effectiveness of nursing outcomes. These are highlighted by Jones and Mullee (1995), who were unable to demonstrate statistical evidence of different outcomes for patients between nurse-run asthma care and traditional approaches. This emphasises the necessity for nurses to develop tools with which to clarify and measure the outcomes of their interventions.

It is also possible that nurse-led clinics may lead to greater costs because nurses engaged in the delivery of holistic care frequently discover more needs in their patients. An example of this was found in the enuresis clinic. It was clear to the nurse leading the clinic that the parents of some children were either intolerant of the problem or overprotective of their children. They suffered from guilt, blaming themselves for a lack of parenting skills. It was felt that the situation could be improved by helping to promote simple positive parenting skills and evaluating the results. However, this has time and resource implications for an already overstretched service. Having uncovered a problem, the financial situation can make it difficult to resolve within a health service setting.

In conclusion, some examples of an evolving field of paediatric ambulatory nursing have been explored and the benefits and problems highlighted. Questions need to asked about the future of this nursing role. The successful outcome of the Southampton enuresis clinic and some of the others mentioned here has implications for the introduction of more nurse-led clinics. In the present climate, where medical staff are under much pressure to perform to given targets, there is no better time for a nurse to identify unmet needs in the ambulatory care of the child and family and, with medical and managerial support, to expand their roles in order to provide a quality service.

As more and more nurses in the UK embark upon Master's degree programmes, it is likely that higher education will release as yet untapped nursing creativity, confidence and entrepreneurism. It may be that nurses will develop more conviction about their place as equal partners with the medical profession in the delivery of high-quality health care to children and their families. Some nurses may wish to exercise more autonomy and develop as paediatric nurse practitioners on the lines of their US counterparts, holding open clinics for children with undiagnosed problems.

The current climate of economic austerity can be advantageous to nursing innovation, as has been demonstrated in the USA (Stilwell, 1988). However, in order to exploit the potential of such innovations, it is vital that paediatric nursing has influence on purchasers and providers. This will ensure that paediatric nursing is offered as a high-quality, cost-effective service that can be purchased by consortia alongside medical care to meet differing patient needs (RCN, 1993).

Clearly, evidence of cost-effectiveness and of high-quality nursing outcomes must be provided. Thus a vital future step is to develop suitable research methodologies and gain funding for large-scale studies to evaluate whether nursing interventions are improving patient outcomes. However, it is clear that, within a rapidly changing health care environment such as exists today, there are many challenges and opportunities for paediatric nurses to develop holistic ambulatory care for children in the new millennium.

References

Angeli, N., Christy, J., Howe, J. and Wolff, B. (1994) Facilitating parenting skills in vulnerable families. *Health Visitor*, **67**(4): 130–2.

Bradbury, M. and Meadow, S.R. (1995) Combined treatment with enuresis alarm and desmopressin for noctural enuresis. *Acta Paediatrica*, **84**: 1014–18.

Butler, R. (1994) *Nocturnal Enuresis – the Child's Experience*. (Oxford: Butterworth Heinemann).

Butterworth, T. (1991) Setting our professional house in order, in Salvage, J. (ed.) *Nurse Practitioners: Working for Change in Primary Health Care Nursing*. (London: King's Fund Centre).

Callery, P. (1997) Using evidence in children's nursing. *Paediatric Nursing,* **9**(6): 13–17.

Castledine, G. (1993) Nurses should welcome a wider scope of practice. *British Journal of Nursing,* **2**(13): 686–7.

Clark, G., Fleming, C., Hable, A. *et al.* (1994) Nocturnal enuresis: a strategy for management. Produced for Ferring Pharmaceuticals, Feltham, Middlesex.

Evans, A. and Griffiths, P. (1994) *The Development of a Nursing-led In-patient Service.* (London: King's Fund Centre).

Hampson, G.D. (1994) *Bolden and Takle's Practice Nurse Handbook.* (Oxford: Blackwell Scientific).

International Council of Nurses (1992) *Guidelines on 'Specialisation in Nursing.* (Geneva: ICN).

Jones, K.P. and Mullee, M. (1995) Proactive, nurse-run asthma care in general practice reduces asthma morbidity: scientific fact or medical assumption? *British Journal of General Practice,* **45**: 497–9.

Kempe, C. and Helfer, R. (1972) *Helping the Battered Child and his Family.* (Oxford: Lippincott).

Kobryn, M. and Pearce, S. (1991) The paediatric nurse practitioner. *Paediatic Nursing,* **3**(5): 11–14.

Madge, P. (1995) Can nursing intervention improve outcome in children hospitalised with acute asthma: a randomised study. *European Respiratory Journal,* **8**(suppl. 19): 11s.

Millar M. and Booth, E. (1996) Health of the young nation: a primary care team approach. *Health Visitor,* **69**(4): 147–8.

NHS Management Executive (1991) *The New Deal.* (London: NHSME).

Palmer, C. (1995) A joint approach to asthma. *Child Health,* **2**(5): 207–10.

Read, S. and Graves, K. (1994) *Reduction of Junior Doctors' Hours in Trent Region: the Nursing Contribution.* Sheffield Centre for Health and Related Research/NHSE Trent.

Rees, M. and Kinnersley, P. (1996) Nurse-led management of minor illness in a general practice surgery. *Nursing Times,* **92**(6): 32–3.

Royal College of Nursing (1993) *The Role of Nurses in Purchasing for Health Gain: RCN Information.* (London: RCN).

Royal College of Nursing (1995) *Clinical Guidelines: What You Need To Know.* (London: Scutari/RCN).

Stilwell, B. (1988) The origins and development of the nurse practitioner role – a worldwide perspective. In Bowling, A. and Stilwell, B. (eds) *The Nurse in Family Practice.* (London: Scutari Press).

Stilwell, B., Greenfield, S., Dinny, M. and Hull, F. (1987) A nurse practitioner in general practice: working style and pattern of consultations. *Journal of the Royal College of GPs,* **37**: 154–7.

Thornes, R. (1993) *Bridging the Gaps.* (London: Action for Sick Children).

UKCC (1994) *The Future of Professional Practice: The Council's Standards for Education and Practice Following Registration.* (London: UKCC).

Wooler, E. (1993) The role of the asthma nurse specialist. *Paediatric Respiratory Medicine,* **1**(2): 26–8.

Wright, S. (1992) Exporting excellence. *Nursing Times,* **88**(39): 40–2.

10

THE ROLE OF THE CLINICAL NURSE SPECIALIST IN THE PROVISION OF PAEDIATRIC AMBULATORY CARE

E.A. Glasper and Susan Lowson

The terms 'clinical nurse specialist', 'consultant nurse' and 'nurse practitioner' are an increasing part of modern nursing nomenclature. Although such terms are used extensively throughout the profession, they are often used interchangeably and, as a result, much confusion surrounds their defined roles. Changes in junior doctors' working hours in the UK, coupled with reprofiled health reforms, have placed nursing in the professional spotlight. Rapid changes in service delivery to patients, linked to a demise of inpatient care and a corresponding rise in ambulatory care, have accelerated the trend towards specialisation within nursing. Castledine (1995) has indicated that the nurse practitioner/specialist movement in the UK may be seen as nothing more than a stopgap for the shortage of doctors. Despite this, the robustness of the movement in North America is such that the American Academy of Nurse Practitioners (1993) believes that nurse practitioners have performed as well as physicians with respect to patient outcomes, proper diagnosis, management of specified medical conditions and frequency of patient satisfaction. American definitions of terms tend to have greater clarity than those used in the UK; for example, the American Academy of Nurse Practitioners defines nurse practitioners as primary health care providers. Although not defined, clinical nurse specialists (CNSs) are seen as hospital based, and the term is therefore useful for those nurses offering a service that effectively operates at the primary/secondary/tertiary interface, that is, ambulatory care.

Although the debate over who or what constitutes a CNS goes on, Ryan has concluded that expert direct care provider, educator, communicator and researcher are all essential ingredients of the post. McGee *et al.* (1996) have shown that recent research has revealed that teaching, clinical practice and working as a consultant/adviser are now the chief activities of the CNS, with management, research and audit being less common.

Paediatric ambulatory care is fertile ground for the evolution of CNSs and, in the wake of *Bridging the Gaps* (Thornes, 1993), it is imperative that services be developed and improved. While the development of the paediatric CNS meets the aspirations of publications such as *Bridging the Gaps*, it also interfaces with the NHS document *A Service with Ambitions* (Department of Health, 1996). Clinical nurse specialism within paediatric ambulatory care has grown to meet the needs of families rather than the professional ambitions of the nurses themselves. A number of examples from the University Hospital in Southampton are offered as CNS models with an ambulatory care perspective.

Genetics

The specialist nurse in genetics in Britain has evolved historically within the development of clinical genetics as a medical speciality. The basis of genetic counselling relies crucially on a firm medical diagnosis. This necessitates the placing of the service within the medical domain. However, accepted definitions of genetic counselling emphasise the educational and support components, describing it as a process that is concerned with diagnosis, the transmission of information about risks of inheriting or passing on a medical problem, and the support of individuals in coming to terms with those risks and in making decisions (Ad Hoc Committee on Genetic Counselling, 1975).

The comprehensive nature of genetic counselling provides an ideal environment for multidisciplinary work.. There is an identified need for genetic counselling co-workers who are genetically literate and fully equipped to meet the educational and counselling needs of the families. In the UK, there is a predominance of nurses within clinical genetic services. This is in contrast to other countries where there are well-established Master's level 'genetic counsellor' training programmes that are open to both nurses and non-nurses.

The role of the genetic CNS has slowly evolved since the appointment of the first UK genetic nurse in 1959, and the number employed has doubled since 1988. The scope of their practice has recently been analysed (Skirton *et al.*, 1995), and the role of the nurse in facilitating the process of genetic counselling is similar to that of genetic counsellors. However, it appears that the nurses and associates that responded to the more recent survey are increasingly holding their own caseload of clients and providing genetic counselling. It was emphasised that the ideal approach is that of a team and where a combination of a medical and nursing model of care allows for a sharing of strengths of all members of the team and ensures adequate patient care and autonomy.

An examination of the membership of the UK Association of Genetic Nurses and Counsellors shows that 91 per cent are registered nurses, the majority having additional post-registration qualifications such as health visiting or midwifery. Approximately 24 per cent of the nurses in Skirton's study had completed or were currently studying at Master's level, and the average length of experience in clinical genetics was 6 years (range 7 months to 15 years). This may suggest that the nurses already in post are identifying their own educational requirements, which may be at postgraduate level. It may also suggest a considerable reliance on the development of expertise through the synthesis of practical experience within the speciality.

The expansion of clinical genetics in the past 10 years has meant an expansion in the number of personnel employed within the service. This expansion means that the nurse or co-worker has to define her role and models of practice clearly in order to maintain her own individual contribution to client care (Tinley, 1987). For nurses, the changes in post-registration levels of practice and education also require an acknowledgement and maintenance of their professional standards (UKCC, 1992). Although the individuals and the setting in which they work strongly influence the development of their role, the location of the practice within the profession of nursing requires a broader base to ensure adherence to professional norms.

Epilepsy

The role of the paediatric epilepsy nurse specialist (PENS) is clearly accepted by many paediatric neurologists and paediatricians. However, the number of PENSs in the UK is very small. Indeed, the number of epilepsy nurse specialists (ENSs) working across all age groups has only recently reached double figures in the UK.

The role of the PENS at Southampton University Hospital grew out of the role of the paediatric neurology liaison nurse. Children under the care of the paediatric neurologists often have chronic conditions requiring complex treatment regimens. In 1994, it was identified by the paediatric neurologists and the existing paediatric neurology liaison nurse that children with epilepsy and their families would benefit from a different model of care. Such a model would promote holistic care and be facilitated through the appointment of a CNS. It was decided that the existing liaison nurse should be helped to develop her role to become the nurse specialist. Another nurse was subsequently employed to fulfil the liaison role. In order to develop the new model, guidance and advice were sought from other UK children's units. It was anticipated that the CNS would carry his or her own individual caseload, and a cohort of families was identified from those attending the paediatric neurology outpatients clinics. In addition, a protocol was developed in which family health care physicians were requested to refer newly diagnosed children with epilepsy to the PENS. Aird *et al.* (1984) have indicated that the ultimate aim of any treatment for epilepsy is to help the sufferer to achieve satisfactory life adjustment. This might entail the provision of continuing emotional support and education for an indefinite period.

Epilepsy affects 1 in 100 children, 75 per cent of people with epilepsy being diagnosed before the age of 20. This is clearly a major childhood concern. There are multiple causes of epilepsy including meningitis, encephalitis, head injury and brain tumour, but the cause remains unknown in 50–70 per cent of cases. A diagnosis of epilepsy can have a devastating effect on the life of the child and can be the cause of major disruptions of family dynamics. The role of the PENS is to support the child and family during the first few months following diagnosis and continue this contact until the child is transferred to adult care professionals. Education and advice for schools, employers, friends and relatives can help to ensure that the child receives a non-discriminatory transition through childhood.

The benefits of this service are considerable, ranging from an improved monitoring of the control of the epilepsy in an individual child to liaison with schools and community-based personnel, and the organisation of support groups for families of children with epilepsy (Appleton, 1993).

The specialist nurse is hospital based within a child health directorate. The nurse attends weekly epilepsy clinics, together with the paediatric neurologist, to provide information, support and advice. Liaison takes place with children with epilepsy who are inpatients and their families, and between the hospital, community and school personnel. This nurse acts as a point of first contact for parents who are able to telephone for advice related to their child's medication and seizure control, in addition to concerns regarding daily living. An extensive range of information leaflets, drug information sheets, books and ideas on all aspects of epilepsy is available from the nurse specialist. The PENS is also involved in standard-setting, audit, quality of life studies and clinical trials.

The introduction of a nurse-led clinic provides a further setting for parents/carers to discuss concerns not necessarily related to medication changes. The nurse specialist is thus able to co-ordinate additional services required by the family in the community.

In 1990 the cost to the UK Health Service for each person with epilepsy was £600 in the year in which diagnosis was made, this figure falling to less than £200 in subsequent years when seizures were well controlled (Cockerell et al., 1994). However, the cost of social services was five to ten times higher, depending on the frequency of seizures. Better care and fewer seizures might therefore lead to a net gain for both patients and society (Ridsdale, 1995). The provision of specialist ambulatory care and the utilisation of the PENS might, therefore, be seen as prudent in a climate of financial austerity. The continuing education of nurses specialising in the field of epilepsy is available in the form of a certificate in the care of people with epilepsy, a diploma in epilepsy care and a Master's degree in Epileptology. The formation of the Epilepsy Specialist Nurses Association (ESNA) and the initiation in 1995 of the British Epilepsy Association Sapphire Nurse Scheme should ensure that this group of nurses will continue to thrive.

Sapphire nurse scheme

This is a joint venture by the British Epilepsy Association and Glaxo-Wellcome, a major pharmaceutical company, to fund 16 ENS posts for 2 years.

Diabetes

Insulin-dependent diabetes is one of the most common chronic disorders of childhood (Dorman *et al.*, 1995). A UK national survey carried out in 1988 (Metcalfe and Baum, 1991) showed that the incidence of childhood-onset diabetes had nearly doubled in the previous decade to 13.5 for every 100000 children per year. Murphy (1994) cites Ludvigsson (1991), who suggests that children with diabetes should be cared for by a multidisciplinary team with a specialised knowledge of diabetes in children. This team should include a paediatric diabetes nurse specialist.

In a study related to the nursing care of children with diabetes, Moyer (1993) describes the historical development of the specialist role that began with the introduction of a specialised health visiting service more than 50 years ago. Walker (1953) evaluates the Leicester specialised health visiting service for children and adults with diabetes as showing demonstrable benefits to patients. These benefits included a decreased admission to hospital for ketoacidosis, an increased attendance at clinic, improved self-care and enhanced feelings of well-being. Challen *et al.* (1990) highlight the importance of the specialist nurse/health visitor in the care of adults and children. Following a psychological survey of young people with diabetes, which included an investigation of the views of parents and the support received from hospital, Challen conclude that the provision of a diabetic health visitor service would improve the support to families of children with diabetes.

McEvilly (1995) describes how the role of the paediatric diabetes specialist nurse differs from the role of the adult specialist nurse. In particular, the need for family-centred care to be adjusted to the changing needs of the individual child and family is important. In 1993, because of concern about the increasing numbers of children with diabetes, the Royal College of Nursing Paediatric Diabetes Special Interest Group established a working party to identify the roles and qualifications required for nurses giving care and support to children with diabetes and their families.

The Royal College of Nursing working party report identified several key areas in the role of the paediatric diabetes CNS:

- identifying needs and facilitating the implementation of services
- the organisation and management of personnel, services and resources
- a small clinical caseload

- setting standards, developing quality management and audit to include the provision of appropriate protocols
- the provision of appropriate diabetes education for patients, families, carers, the public and nursing, medical and other professionals
- the development of teamwork by the identification of roles and common aims
- initiating nursing research and development programmes
- extending and utilising counselling skills
- continuing personal development by participation in the current activities of professional bodies
- professional accountability according to the UKCC Code of Conduct.

The report provides a framework within which it is hoped services for children with diabetes will continue to develop. The report also suggests that the peripatetic role of the paediatric diabetes specialist nurse should enable her to develop closer relationships with families that would be otherwise impossible to achieve in a tertiary clinical setting.

The Royal College of Nursing working party recommends that all nurses caring for children with diabetes should hold paediatric, community and diabetes qualifications. The English National Board 928 certificate course in diabetes nursing has provided basic diabetes nurse training since 1982, and diploma and degree-level courses in diabetes care have recently been established. The ENB 928 course includes a component on childhood diabetes. However, to date, there has not been a recognised, accredited course in paediatric diabetes nursing, although Birmingham Children's Hospital runs a course in the management of childhood diabetes for nurses and dietitians.

When setting up such a specialist service, wide discussion is required not only with paediatricians and managers, but also with regional referral centres to establish their needs. Close liaison with community colleagues, particularly health visitors, is essential to ensure their appreciation of the role and full understanding that it will enhance their role rather than rival it.

Cystic fibrosis

The development of specialist centres providing treatment for cystic fibrosis (CF) patients coupled with the increasing use of home intravenous antibiotic therapy are probably the two main contributory factors in the evolution of the CF CNS. CF remains the most common serious pulmonary and genetic disease of children, although the life expectancy for sufferers has markedly improved in recent years. The success of modern therapy linked to the growth in CF nurse specialists is now ensuring greater longevity and quality of life for CF children. The UK's first CF CNS was appointed at the Brompton Hospital in London in 1980 (cited in Dyer, 1991), and the success of this first post has resulted in a steady growth throughout the country. Each post is unique in that the nurses fulfil their own unique role among their patient group. Although each post differs in terms of job description, there are areas common to all. Dyer (1991) has suggested that the following principles underpin the role of the CF nurse specialist:

- clinical support
- patient support
- education
- liaison and information resource
- patient advocacy.

Clinical support primarily involves the teaching, assessment and monitoring of procedures carried out at home. In the past, these would have been undertaken in hospital with the parents/child as passive bystanders during the inpatient stay. The growth of ambulatory care has considerably reduced the need for hospital admission and, with CNS support, families are able to consider enteral feeding, the administration of intravenous antibiotics and other therapies. As a consequence, the need for hospital admission has been greatly reduced. In addition, the increasing emphasis on care in the community has ensured that therapies that were once considered to be possible only in hospital can now be given at home. This has led to an increased demand by families for interventions that avoid an inpatient stay. The role of the CF CNS is essential in ensuring that such treatments are administered appropriately and are beneficial to patients and their families. The ambulatory and home management of children with CF can offer many advantages but only when appropriately supported by nursing staff.

Patient support is carried out within the multidisciplinary team, which in some centres includes a psychologist and a social worker. In centres that do not have a full complement of practitioners, it is the CNS who takes a primary role in these areas. In Southampton, this support by the CNS begins from diagnosis and extends to terminal care and bereavement follow-up. In working closely with families, the CF specialist nurse is able to gain insight into how they function as a unit, sharing in the highs as well as the lows.

The growth in the number of children who are surviving well into adult life has challenged paediatric nurses in that there are now many occasions when patients have to be handed on to an adult-focused team of professionals. What was once a rarity is now commonplace. It is, however, difficult for nurses who have cared for these children since birth to pass them on to other colleagues, and this is perhaps a tribute to the growing professionalism of the nursing profession as a whole.

The educational element of the CF CNS role is focused primarily on the child and family as an indivisible unit and is clearly dictated by the age of the patient and his or her level of overall development. In addition to the educative supportive role of the nurse to the child and family is that of education given to other professional staff who come into contact with the family.

The regular updating of medical and nursing staff *vis-à-vis* recent developments in the care of CF patients plays a major role in ensuring the highest standards of patient care. The nurse specialist also has a role in providing education to those other individuals who come into contract on a regular basis with CF patients. These include school, college and club personnel. Ignorance and fear of the unknown can lead to unnecessary restrictions being placed on the child. The utilisation of informed open evenings and so on can provide a valuable opportunity for the nurse specialist to interact with such contacts, leading to the exchange of ideas and the clarification of misconceptions.

The liaison and information-giving role of nurse specialists is considerable and is one of their most important functions. The vast array of medical and social contacts that CF families have makes this particular role vital, the nurse specialist acting pivotally in bridging the gaps between the primary/secondary and tertiary areas of medical care. In ensuring consistent management, the CNS effectively prevents confusion arising in the delivery of patient care.

Patient advocacy for this type of client is perceived to be an extremely important aspect of the CF CNS. As treatment continues to advance, new hopes and fears are engendered within patients and their families. It is, therefore, vital that CNSs are able to adapt and help the families to cope throughout the difficult periods of their lives.

Nephrology

The role of the nephrology CNS within ambulatory care is expanding as the frontiers of medicine push forward the ability of families to manage renal disease in the home environment. The decline of hospital-based programmes is allowing an ambulatory care investment that effectively manages children at home or in an outpatients department. The ability to manage children utilising home peritoneal dialysis is attributed to the expertise of the nephrology CNSs. Establishing peritoneal dialysis at home requires home assessment and the extensive education of local and community professionals involved with their care. The CNSs. have developed comprehensive guidelines and discharge planners to ensure continuing high standards of care and safety in the home situation.

The establishment of a renal outpatients clinic that is jointly run by the CNS and the nephrologist is seen as particularly innovative. The production of an education/information resource for newly diagnosed children and their families is available in both verbal and booklet format.

Neonatal surgery

The development of the neonatal family care nurse specialist (NFCS) has evolved through the recognition that families need substantial support when they require the services of a surgical neonatal intensive care unit. This begins in the antenatal period when screening may have revealed an anatomical defect that requires surgical intervention after birth.

The NFCS is present at the first consultation with the family at the antenatal stage. This allows the nurse to begin preparation of the family for the journey ahead. This may entail the communication with a range of health care professionals and possibly introducing the family to other families who have lived through similar situations.

It must be appreciated that the ability of families in such circumstances to make decisions is seriously compromised. At times, this becomes almost impossible for families as they struggle to cope with getting from day to day. The role of the specialist nurse in providing information and support is important in helping families to become aware of options and choices that may be open to them. The ability of the NFCS to support families from diagnosis to discharge and then provide a plan of continued care in the community effectively enhances self-esteem and shifts the locus of control from professional to family.

NFCSs work in all settings to maintain their clinical skills. It is vital to preserve clinical competence to ensure that the knowledge and ability to appreciate the needs of the child and family do not deteriorate.

The continuing role of the paediatric CNS in ambulatory care

Clinical nurse specialism is not a new phenomenon. The growth of ambulatory care as a discrete discipline in its own right is perhaps fertile ground for the continuing growth of the nurse specialist. There is no doubt that family advocacy is one of the key aspects of the paediatric CNS role. This entails a close relationship with the family, and the role will only be successful when this occurs. Voicing the views of the child and the family does not always make the specialist nurse popular among colleagues, but that should not deter them in their quest to improve standards of care.

As a consequence, specialist nurses must be articulate about their role and the effectiveness of their work. This will entail the maintenance of data on clinical outcomes, for these nurses have to exist in a world dominated by evidence-based care. Although much has been written on the role of the CNS, it will be for paediatric nurse specialists to effectively underpin their own roles with the appropriate educational and vocational courses. New clinical Master's degrees will help to give these nurses the legitimacy they will need in the future. Ambulatory care is an area wide open for nursing innovation. It is hoped that paediatric nurses around the world will respond positively to this challenge.

Acknowledgements

Our thanks go to Christine Patch (genetics), Alison Fielder (epilepsy), Heather Murphy (diabetes), Carolyn Redman (family support), Maggie Randall (nephrology), Judi Maddison (cystic fibrosis) – six specialist nurses who impress us greatly and are all challenging the way in which children are cared for.

References

Ad Hoc Committee on Genetic Counselling (1975) in Genetic counselling, *American Journal of Human Genetics*, **27**: 240–2.

Aird, R.A., Masland, R.L. and Woodbury, D.M. (1984) *The Epilepsies. A Critical Review.* (New York: Raven Press).

American Academy of Nurse Practitioners (1993) *Standards of Practice.* (American Academy of Nurse Practitioners).

Appleton, R. (1993) Special link… why the clinical nurse specialist for children with epilepsy is urgently required. *Nursing Times*, **89**(19): 40–1.

Castledine, G. (1995) Will the nurse practitioner be a mini-doctor or a maxi-nurse? *British Journal of Nursing*, **4**(16): 938–9.

Challen, A.H., Davies, A.G., Williams, R.J.W. and Baum, J.D. (1990) Support for families with diabetic children: parents' views. *Practical Diabetes*, **7**(1): 26–31.

Cockerell, D., Hart, Y.M., Sander, J.W.A.S. and Shorvon, S.D. (1994) The cost of epilepsy in the United Kingdom: an estimation based on the results of two population-based studies. *Epilepsy Research*, **18**: 249–60.

Department of Health (1996) *The National Health Service: A Service with Ambitions.* (London: HMSO).

Dorman, J.S., O'Leary, L.A. and Koehler, A.N. (1995) Epidemiology of childhood diabetes, in Kelnar, C.J.H. (ed.) *Childhood and Adolescent Diabetes.* (London: Chapman & Hall, p. 139).

Dyer, J. (1991) *The Role of the Cystic Fibrosis Nurse Specialist*, Glaxo meeting. (London).

Ludvigsson, J. (1991) Progress report on care of diabetic children and adolescents. *Diabetes in the Young*, **27**: 10–11.

McEvilly, A. (1995) Liaison nursing – the diabetic home care team, in Kelnar, C.J.H. (ed.) *Childhood and Adolescent Diabetes.* (London: Chapman & Hall, pp. 465–73).

McGee, P., Castledine, G. and Brown, R. (1996) A survey of specialist and advanced nursing practice in England. *British Journal of Nursing*, **5**(11): 682–6.

Metcalfe, M. and Baum, D.J. (1991) Incidence of insulin dependent diabetes in children under 15 years in the British Isles during 1988. *British Medical Journal*, **302**: 443–7.

Moyer, A.A. (1993) The specialist nursing care of children with diabetes. DPhil thesis, University of London.

Murphy, H. (1994) Diabetes in childhood. *British Journal of Nursing*, **3**(17): 892–6.

Ridsdale, L. (1995) Matching the needs with skills in epilepsy care. *British Medical Journal*, **310**: 1219–20.

Ryan, S. (1996) Defining the role of the specialist nurse. *Nursing Standard*, **10**(17): 27–9.

Skirton, H., Barnes, C., Curtis, G. and Walford-Moore, J. (1997) The role and practice of the genetic nurse: report of the AGMC Working Party. *Journal of Medical Genetics*, **34**(2): 141–7.

Thornes, R. (1993) *Bridging the Gaps: Caring for Children in the Health Services. An Exploratory Study of the Interfaces between Primary and Specialist Care for Children within the Health Services.* (London: Action for Sick Children).

Tinley, S.T. (1987) Nurses' and geneticists' role expectations for the genetics nurse clinician. *Journal of Pediatric Nursing: Nursing Care of Children and Families*, **2**(4): 259–64.

UKCC (1992) *The Scope of Professional Practice.* (London: UKCC).

Walker, J.B. (1953) Field work of a diabetic clinic. *Lancet*, **2**: 445–7.

11

THE ROLE OF THE COMMUNITY CHILDREN'S NURSE IN ENHANCING THE PRIMARY–SECONDARY CARE INTERFACE

Paulajean Kelly

Introduction

Paediatric care in the 1990s can be characterised by relatively short hospital admissions and increasing numbers of acute and chronically sick children requiring care at home (Department of Health, 1991; Lessing and Tatman, 1991). As the contributors to this book indicate, developments in paediatric nursing and medicine have not only increased the numbers of children surviving with complex and serious conditions, but have also led to the delivery of care in a much wider variety of settings. This changing pattern has highlighted the need to focus on the relationship between hospital and community care for children (Thornes, 1993).

Central to any discussion on the interface between primary and secondary services in paediatrics is the provision and adequate resourcing of a community children's nursing service. These services provide specialist paediatric care in the community, giving families support in caring for their sick child at home. They provide additional resources to families that complement the community nursing services of health visiting and school nursing, whose focus and expertise is child health and general practitioner services, with their responsibility for the medical health of the whole family. These teams employ nurses with training and experience in community and paediatric nursing, and therefore occupy an ideal position for interfacing with hospital nursing and medical staff, and with members of the primary health care team to ensure continuity of care.

Information exchange is at the core of interfacing between services, and although detailed information about complex and changing management regimens is essential to parents caring for a sick child at home, there is a debate on the control of information exchange between professionals. This may have the potential to delay access to services that, under the current Health Service reforms, will be increasingly community led and managed (Community Care Act 1990). Failure to recognise this ignores the role of the primary health care team in continuing to address other health care issues that will affect the child and family, in addition to their diagnosis of a chronic or acute illness that requires 'paediatric' intervention.

In seeking to explore these issues, the chapter will highlight the 'interface' between services through an examination of the processes and structures that exist to support this dialogue and an evaluation of the efficacy of those structures to meet the needs of both clients and professionals. Clinical case histories indicated that there is a need for flexibility in provision and to continually review the balance between support and practical help for families.

Historical development of community children's nursing

The first services were developed in the UK in the early and mid-1950s in Rotherham (Gillett, 1954), Paddington in London (Lightwood, 1956) and Birmingham (Smellie, 1956). The Rotherham service was established in response to a prolonged outbreak of gastroenteritis in the city, severely straining hospital inpatient bed resources. This set a theme in the establishment and operation of community children's nursing services of meeting the specific needs of a local community that persists today. How these needs are defined may vary in relation to a specific disease process, geography and other physical resources such as the number of paediatric inpatient beds.

The rationale behind the provision of these early and subsequent services is that hospitals as a form of institutional care can be emotionally and psychologically damaging to children (Bowlby, 1965; Hawthorn, 1974; Robertson and Robertson, 1989). Successive government reports (Ministry of Health, 1959; Department of Health, 1976, 1991, 1996a, 1996b; Audit Commission, 1993) have advocated an expansion in services providing nursing care for sick children in settings other than inpatient wards.

Despite their recommendations, the growth in the number of and size of services has been slow and characterised by short bursts of expansion, particularly during the late 1980s and early 1990s (Whiting 1988; Whiting et al., 1994; Royal College of Nursing, 1995). Explanations for this slow and at times negligible growth would require a detailed analysis of the economic, health care and philo-sophical issues confronting child health and its location within the NHS and are outside the remit of this chapter.

It is interesting to note within a volume concerned with innova-tive ways of developing health care for children two issues that may be of relevance, since these correlate positively with the develop-ment of community children's nursing services. First, expansions in existing services and the creation of new services have been funded from a variety of sources that include the closure of paediatric wards in smaller hospitals as a result of an overall decentralisation of hospital services (Jennings, 1994). Central government has under-written funding initiatives to support particularly vulnerable groups of children (While et al., 1995) and an expansion in the provi-sion of community children's nursing posts has been sponsored through the charity sector (Hunt, 1995).

Second, there has been a shift in emphasis for paediatric nursing professionals and pressure groups concerned with the welfare of sick children, from the care and welfare of hospitalised children to a concern with children's health experiences wherever they occur (Thornes, 1993). The relationship between available funding to develop new services and lobbying activities of professionals and voluntary organisations, combined with organisational changes in the NHS, although complex, is particularly important when consid-ering the role that community children's nurses play in negotiating between different service stakeholders in providing care for sick children in the home.

Current roles of community children's nurses

There are currently 149 general and specialist services operating within the UK (Royal College of Nursing, 1995). National research carried out in the early 1990s indicated either that a considerable number of children lived in an area where no service existed or that the level of service was difficult to predict because of the size and scope of teams varying so widely (Tatman and Woodroffe, 1993). This chapter is focused on the role of the generalist community children's nursing services. These services are likely to restrict their area to a community Trust and/or all paediatric patients seen by a particular hospital Trust, depending on local purchasing and providing contracts (Royal College of Nursing, 1993). The wide variety in provision may range from large community-orientated teams of nurses providing a comprehensive range of services, including evening and weekend visiting, to smaller teams or even individual nurses who are likely to prioritise children with complex chronic conditions, usually on a hospital outreach basis (Kelly et al., 1995). The latter half of the 1990s has also seen the introduction of more acutely orientated services to support ambulatory assessment units in A&E departments (Brown and Penna, 1996; Gallagher, 1996).

Given the improvements in the nature of hospital care for sick children and the reduction in average length of stay (Henderson et al., 1991), does the argument for a service to provide care at home remain as strong as it was in the 1950s? Recent research has indicated (Callery and Smith, 1991; Darbyshire, 1994; Callery, 1997) that hospitalisation remains problematic for children and their families, as this graphic comment by a parent of a child in hospital indicates:

When you are in hospital you are living in somebody else's work space (Tatman et al., 1992).

In addition, advances in medicine and nursing have changed the profile of many acute and chronic disorders for children (Henderson et al., 1992), increasing rather than reducing the need for home follow-up.

The objectives of community children's nursing services can be summarised as:

1. *Prevention of hospital admission*
   The primary health care team, paediatric outpatients and A&E departments can refer children with acute and chronic conditions for management at home rather than admitting them to hospital.

2. *Shortening of hospital admission*
   Children can be discharged home earlier, and their nursing care continued at home once they are over the most acute phase of their illness. Practical nursing care can be given by the commu-

nity children's nurses through intermittent home visits, working with families who, in addition to having overall care for their child, may learn specialised nursing techniques themselves.

3. *Prevention of readmission*

Monitoring children with chronic illnesses in their own environment at home, and older children at school, not only provides a more accurate picture of their condition than a short hospital outpatients appointment, but may also result in nursing staff being alerted earlier to changes in their condition. Interventions at this stage can prevent the child requiring a hospital admission. In addition, supporting families of chronically sick children may alleviate some of the emotional and psychological pressures on families that can in some circumstances precipitate hospital admission.

4. *The provision of specialist nursing advice*

The services are able to provide paediatric nursing advice to health care professionals in the community to support them in managing the care of sick children at home. Hospital paediatric services can access information about several aspects of caring for a sick child at home, thereby facilitating discharge planning. Finally, this experience and expertise in caring for sick children at home is also available to parents. Providing education about treatment regimens or specific aspects of their child's management in hospital or at home, in a setting within which the family is likely to feel most comfortable and in control, is likely to have several advantages.

Children and their families can therefore be appropriately referred to a community children's nursing service by a wide range of health care professionals in the hospital and community. Those referred have a wide variety of health care needs, some with acute short-term problems and others with conditions requiring longer-term management and support.

They include children with common chronic conditions such as asthma and eczema. Teaching children and their families about the disease process for these conditions enables them to understand more clearly the rationale of treatment, which may improve compliance. Thus using a home nebuliser or other inhaler device can be set within the context of the child's overall care, and parents can gain skills and confidence in the assessment and management of the condition, knowing in which circumstances to seek further medical advice (Childs and Dezateux, 1991).

More detailed knowledge about the chronic nature of a condition such as eczema can help families to adapt topical treatment regimens for the child's maximum benefit. Teaching parents the principles of management in a supportive environment at home with easy access to further advice can result in conditions such as eczema being successfully managed at home and children rarely requiring admission, even for acute exacerbations (Tatman *et al.*, 1992). Children who require dressings post-surgery, or after minor trauma such as burns and scalds, can be treated in their own homes, a much more comforting environment than a hospital ward or A&E department.

Premature babies can be discharged home earlier, the extra support they need from nasogastric feeding or in some cases low-flow oxygen being managed by their families with support from the community children's nursing service (Southall and Samuels, 1990). Children with a wide range of stomas, including tracheostomies, ileostomies, colostomies and gastrostomies, can be discharged home early and then supported in giving their nursing care at home. A whole range of nursing care can be given safely at home by parents supported by a community children's nursing service, including the administration of intravenous therapy (Evans, 1994).

Other conditions, such as nephrotic syndrome, hydronephrosis, congenital heart disease and haemoglobinopathies, can be monitored at home, reducing the need for hospital outpatients and day case attendances. This is particularly important when we consider that children with these conditions will inevitably spend a considerable time in hospital. Children with cancer can be monitored at home following chemotherapy, and support can be provided in reintegrating them back into school (Bignold *et al.*, 1994). For children with life-threatening and life-limiting conditions, the community children's nurse would aim to meet their families as early as possible in their illness trajectory and establish a relationship with the whole family in order that the care provided can be tailored to meet the needs of the individual family (Kelly *et al.*, 1996). If the child requires palliative care, the family have an informed choice about the support they will receive if they wish to nurse their child at home in the final stages of his or her life (Goldman *et al.*, 1990). Community children's nursing services can provide symptom control and co-ordinate respite and bereavement care.

The impact of increasing the life expectations of children with life-limiting illnesses is therefore no longer confined to hospital-based paediatric services (Kelly *et al.*, 1995). Parents have taken on the responsibility of providing complex nursing care in the home setting. Children themselves participate in their care and take on aspects of practical management, for example intermittent catheterisation and the management of central venous lines. The world of the child extends beyond the home setting, and providing appropriate support to enable children to achieve their developmental potential through educational and leisure activities is part of the co-ordinating role of community children's nursing services.

Community children's nurses at the interface

Interfacing with hospital services

The majority of referrals to community children's nurses are from hospital services, either inpatient or outpatient, and therefore most children will be under the care of a paediatrician. The relationship between the community children's nurses and hospital services is the key to the effective co-ordination of caring for sick children at home. Hospital services require a clear understanding of the scope of community children's nursing in order to enable them to make appropriate referrals. Regular meetings between staff from each service are hence essential. These can take a variety of forms including:

- attendance on ward rounds
- participating in outpatient clinics
- attendance at meetings designed to discuss the social and psychological needs of patients and families.

Newly established community children's nursing services need to help hospital staff adjust to a new concept of management and gain trust in the skills of the community nursing team (Tatman *et al.*, 1992). In large teams, individual community children's nurses are able to take responsibility for liaison with a particular ward area, department or speciality; although time-consuming, this regular liaison is vital in maintaining a high level of understanding of roles and skills, and therefore continuity for patients. Many hospital paediatric units have a training function for nursing and medical staff. This, coupled with relatively high staff turnover in the health care professions, increases the need for liaison processes and structures to be ongoing. Regular contact facilitates opportunities for hospital staff to discuss potential referrals and the community children's nurses to meet the families and children who are being referred for follow-up at home. These verbal meetings and discussions need to be supplemented by the exchange of written information, in the form of a written referral from the hospital service to the community children's nurses detailing relevant demographic, social, medical and nursing information about the child and family. For the family, an information leaflet explaining the organisation and purpose of the community children's nursing service and naming the nurse who will be caring for their child at home should be made available (Department of Health, 1996a). The expertise of community children's nursing lies with the sick child and his or her family, and although promoting health in the widest sense is obviously part of their remit, the hospital services need to be aware of the boundary between their work and that of the primary health care team.

Some of these issues can be illustrated by the following case history.

CASE STUDY 1

The neonatal unit at a large inner city teaching hospital manages babies born to women from a wide geographical catchment area. The community children's nursing service based in the local community Trust accepts referrals from the unit for babies requiring long-term nursing care at home. One of the nurses from the team attends the weekly psychosocial meetings on the unit. This is a multidisciplinary meeting including medical and nursing staff from the neonatal unit, the liaison health visitor, paediatric social workers, psychologists and the child psychiatrist. At meetings, all of the babies on the unit are discussed, relating their medical progress to social circumstances. Potential referrals to the team can therefore be highlighted. This case history relates to a baby boy who was referred to the community children's nursing service aged 3 months when it became clear that he had bronchopulmonary dysphasia (Northway, 1990) and would require long-term oxygen therapy.

He was born at 23 weeks gestation, the first child of Nigerian parents who had been living in the UK for the past 6 years. Prior to his birth, both parents were in full-time employment. The mother and father lived together in a privately rented flat on the fourth floor of a block with no lift access and sharing their accommodation with another family who were smokers. On receiving the referral, the community children's nurse organised a preliminary discharge planning meeting. This provided an opportunity for staff from the hospital and community, and the child's parents, to meet together and discuss how his discharge could be organised.

Unsuitable housing emerged as potential delay to discharge and required co-ordinated efforts between the hospital social worker and local authority housing officers to help the parents in applying for more suitable accommodation. The fire services are reluctant for oxygen to be installed above the third floor for safety reasons, and since portable oxygen cylinders are heavy and cumbersome, it is essential to have a lift to enable families to maximise the opportunities for going out. While the family were waiting to be allocated appropriate housing, the community children's nurse took the opportunity to develop a relationship with the parents and explain how the service would aim to support them in caring for their child at home, including the home visiting routine and how to contact the team out of routine office hours via a pager system. The parents were offered the opportunity to meet another family who had taken a child home on low-flow oxygen, which proved very useful to them. Equipment required for home discharge, such as pulse oximeters and portable oxygen cylinders, was demonstrated, and the family were taught infant resuscitation (Angell, 1991).

Arrangements were made with the family's general practitioner for oxygen and other medications to be prescribed and dispensed via a local community pharmacy. For a child who has spent a prolonged and high-dependency period in hospital, families are likely to have a great deal of trust in the hospital unit, and effecting a transfer of this confidence to the community team requires time, patience and close co-operation with the hospital staff. The community children's nurses and other community staff need to be aware of the experiences to which parents will have been exposed during admission. In the case of this child, a baby of similar gestation had died on the unit during his admission, which had an impact on his parents' perception of his prognosis. This had the potential to increase the family's reluctance to go out once at home. The absence of any close relatives in this country was also a potential for increasing their isolation, restricting opportunities for social contact at home and potential baby-sitters. The family were offered suitable accommodation 2 months after the initial referral and a final date for discharge set 2 weeks later, following the installation of an oxygen concentrator and a period of rooming-in by both parents on the neonatal unit to gain confidence in taking 24-hour responsibility for their child's care and management.

On the day of discharge, the parents were accompanied home by their primary nurse from the community children's service, who, once the family were confidently settled, arranged a follow-up visit later in the day. In the initial period at home, the family were visited intensively, recognising the immense change between a neonatal unit and caring for a child at home. Gradually, in close co-operation with the parents, the frequency and duration of visiting were reduced. Close liaison concerning the child's progress with the neonatologist who saw the child regularly in outpatients allowed a high level of specialist medical supervision, despite the child being at home.

This case history illustrates that discharging a child requiring complex care at home requires careful planning and flexibility. Referral mechanisms need to be clear and include policies for feedback and readmission if required. All of these issues rely on mutual trust and respect between the hospital and community, which need to continue once the child has been discharged to facilitate prompt advice from medical staff who have detailed knowledge about the child.

Interfacing with community services

The organisation of community services over a wider geographical area, compared with being focused on a hospital site and larger numbers of personnel, means that the liaison methods described above would not be appropriate. The essential co-operation between community children's nurses and primary health care teams can, however, be achieved at a general level through regular forum meetings and participation in joint training for individual families and children. Discharge planning meetings, as described above for children with complex needs, and frequent telephone and facsimile contact for all are essential.

Exchange of written information via the parent-held child health record (Macfarlane, 1992) means that parents, children and professionals can have a clear idea of each other's involvement in the child's care. Parents are asked to take this booklet with them to all appointments so that any management changes may be recorded. This written information enables professionals unfamiliar with the child (such as a locum general practitioner or A&E doctor) to have access to a summary of the child's history, relieving parents of the burden of explaining details in what may often be a stressful situation.

CASE STUDY 2

The second case history relates to a 7-year-old boy with adrenoleukodystrophy. This is a life-threatening, X-linked genetic disorder that only occurs in boys, affecting the adrenal gland and the white matter of the nervous system. He is the second child in the family affected, his older brother having died less than a year before this child's disease became symptomatic. The family were referred to the community children's nursing service by the boy's consultant paediatric neurologist following the diagnosis of the first child on symptomatology and his asymptomatic brother via a brain scan. The case history concerns the management of the palliative care phase of the second child's illness, reflecting the need for the co-ordination of multiagency involvement. The first indication that the child was displaying overt symptoms of the disease was a convulsion at home, precipitating a short hospital admission for reassessment. The family circumstances were that the parents were divorced and the child lived with his mother and his uncle in a local authority flat on the second floor of a block with lift access. In planning the child's care, the community children's nurses were obviously concerned to take account of the family's experiences with caring for the older sibling in the final stages of his illness.

The primary nurse allocated to the family co-ordinated the medical and nursing care of the child in whichever setting he was being cared for, at home, in hospital or in school, in order to promote continuity. In addition to close discussion with his mother and the child where appropriate, the nurse also co-ordinated liaison between the other key professionals involved by arranging regular review meetings and keeping in contact by telephone. All professionals and the family were encouraged to write in the special parent-held child health record to keep each other informed. This method gave the family a sense of control, essential with so many agencies involved.

The child experienced a gradual loss of neurological function, including deteriorating vision and eventual blindness, loss of motor function, incontinence of bladder and bowel, loss of swallowing reflex and finally loss of speech and consciousness in the last few hours of life. Anticonvulsant therapy proved effective in keeping his fits to a minimum; however, painful muscle spasm proved a more intractable symptom to manage, requiring a combination of muscle relaxants and opiate analgesia to achieve comfort (Hunt and Burne, 1995).

Prior to his deterioration, the child was in mainstream education. His class teacher felt that the familiar environment of school would be vital to maintaining his quality of life despite his increasing disability. The integration of children with special needs into mainstream education is a cornerstone recommendation of the Warnock Report (Department of Education and Science, 1978). The financial burden of caring for a relative with extra nursing care needs at home is recognised by the state (Sainsbury et al., 1995). The community children's nurses worked closely with the family's local authority social worker in making applications for financial resources to ease the practical burden of caring.

CASE STUDY 3

In this case, as the child's caring needs became greater, for example requiring nasogastric feeding in school, extra funding was provided from a voluntary sector charity. The community children's nurses extended their practical advice and support to the school and the child's other carers. The general practitioner held responsibility for the child's medical management at home and worked closely with the community children's nursing team in providing symptom control and supporting the child's mother and uncle, whom the practice had known for a considerable length of time. In the final few days of the child's life, each team was in regular contact to update on current management, ensuring that the nurse and doctor on call were both fully aware of the situation and the level of involvement of each service.

This case indicates how the multiagency needs of the child were met in a co-ordinated manner that enabled the child's mother to have access to the services she required while maintaining the sense that she had control over the manner in which professionals were involved in the care of her child (Gibson, 1995).

Conclusion

This chapter has described the key role that community children's nurses play in interfacing between primary and secondary care services in supporting families caring for sick children at home. The community children's nurse can be seen as acting as a pivot between the services, influencing the balance of their involvement to draw on the different expertise of each as the needs of the child and family dictate. This may mean reducing the hospital service involvement when the child's condition is stable and encouraging the family to refocus their contact with the primary health care team, while ensuring that these services have sufficient information about the child's condition to support the family (Gow and Campbell, 1996).

It can be appreciated that a high level of flexibility is required to meet the needs of individual families effectively and that achieving a balance is not without tensions. For a child with cancer, how much detail a general practitioner and health visitor will need to know about the clinical management will vary according to the particular treatment protocol, the amount of time the child will spend in hospital and the particular needs of an individual family, for example immunising the sick child's siblings. In addition to time resources, supporting a sick child at home will have other financial implications for services involved, such as in the provision of equipment and supplies (Bisset *et al.*, 1992).

Finally, families themselves will be exposed to making decisions about the levels of responsibility they wish to assume in caring for their child (Lantos and Kohram, 1992). Although community children's services are positively evaluated by parents (Tatman *et al.*, 1992; Jennings, 1994), the changes in emphasis to more care being carried out at home has inevitably increased the burden on families already under considerable strain as a result of the child's ill-health (Beresford, 1995). In the absence of appropriate respite, this can militate against the normalisation of family life achieved by the child being at home (Whyte, 1992; Ray and Richlie, 1993). Community children's nurses have a central part to play in exposing these potential tensions and developing strategies to ensure that services and families work together in a co-ordinated way for the maximum benefit of the child.

References

Angell, C. (1991) Equipment requirements for community based paediatric oxygen treatment. *Archives of Disease in Childhood*, **66**: 755.

Audit Commission (1993) *Children First: A Study of Hospital Services.* (London: HMSO).

Beresford, B. (1995) *Expert Opinions: A National Survey of Parents Caring for Disabled Children.* (London: Policy Press).

Bignold, S., Ball, S. and Cribb, A. (1994) Nursing families with children with cancer: the work of the paediatric oncology outreach nurse specialists. London, King's College: Cancer Relief Macmillan Fund/Department of Health.

Bisset, W.M., Stapelford, P., Long, S., Chamberlain, A., Stokel, B. and Millar, P.J. (1992) Home parental nutrition in chronic intestinal failure. *Archives of Disease in Childhood*, **67**: 109–14.

Bowlby, J. (1965) *Child Care and the Growth of Love.* (Harmondsworth: Penguin).

Browne, G.J. and Penna, A. (1996) Short stay facilities: the future of efficient paediatric emergency services. *Archives of Disease in Childhood*, **74**: 309–13.

Callery, P. (1997) Paying to participate: financial social and personal costs to parents of involvement in their child's care in hospital. *Journal of Advanced Nursing*, **25**: 746–52.

Callery, P. and Smith, L. (1991) A study of the role negotiation between nurses and the parents of hospitalised children. *Journal of Advanced Nursing*, **16**: 1771–81.

Childs, H.J. and Dezateux, C.A. (1991) A national survey of nebuliser use. *Archives of Disease in Childhood*, **66**: 1351–3.

Community Care Act (1990) *Caring for People: Community Care in the Next Decade and Beyond*. (London: HMSO).

Darbyshire, P. (1994) *Living With a Sick Child in Hospital: the Experiences of Parents and Nurses*. (London: Chapman & Hall).

Department of Education and Science (1978) *Report of Committee of Enquiry into Special Educational Needs* (Warnock Report). (London: HMSO).

Department of Health (1976) *Report of the Committee on Child Health Services, Fit for the Future* (Court Report). (London: HMSO).

Department of Health (1991) *Welfare of Children and Young People in Hospital*. (London: HMSO).

Department of Health (1996a) *The Children's Charter. Services for Children and Young People*. (London: HMSO).

Department of Health (1996b) *Child Health in the Community: A Guide to Good Practice*. (London: HMSO).

Evans, M. (1994) An investigation into the feasibility of parental participation in the nursing care of their children. *Journal of Advanced Nursing*, **20**: 477–82.

Gallagher, A. (1996) Ambulatory care in practice. *Paediatric Nursing*, **8**(10): 19–20.

Gillet, J. (1954) Children's nursing unit. *British Medical Journal*, **3**: 685.

Goldman, A., Beardsmore, S. and Hunt, J. (1990) Palliative care for children with cancer – home hospital, or hospice? *Archives of Disease in Childhood*, **65**: 641–3.

Gow, M. and Campbell, S. (1996) Paediatric community nursing: doctors' views. *Professional Nurse*, **11**(6): 365–7.

Hawthorn, P.J. (1974) *Nurse: I Want My Mummy*. (London: Royal College of Nursing).

Henderson, J., Goldacre, M.J. and Griffith, M. (1991) Time spent in hospital by children: trends in the Oxford record linkage study area. *Health Trends*, **4**: 166–9.

Henderson, J., Goldacre, M.J., Fairweather, J.M. and Marcovitch, H. (1992) Conditions accounting for substantial time spent in hospital in children aged 1–14 years. *Archives of Disease in Childhood*, **67**: 83–6.

Hunt, A. and Burne, R. (1995) Medical and nursing problems of children with neurodegenerative disease. *Palliative Medicine*, **9**: 19–26.

Hunt, J.A. (1995) The paediatric oncology community nurse specialist: the influence of employment location and funders on models of practice. *Journal of Advanced Nursing*, **22**: 126–33.

Jennings, P. (1994) Learning through experience: an evaluation of hospital at home. *Journal of Advanced Nursing*, **19**(5): 905–11.

Kelly, P.J., Taylor, C. and Tatman, M.A. (1995) Hospital outreach or community nursing? Paediatric home care. *Child Health*, **2**: 4160–3.

Kelly, P.J., Evans, M., Jordan, A. and Orem, V. (1996) Developing a new method to record care at home for children with cancer: an example of research and practice collaboration in a regional paediatric oncology unit. *European Journal of Cancer Care*, **5**: 26–31.

Lantos, J.D. and Kohram, A.F. (1992) Ethical aspects of paediatric home care. *Paediatrics*, **89**: 920–4.

Lessing, D. and Tatman, M.A. (1991) Paediatric home care in the 1990s. *Archives of Disease in Childhood*, **66**: 994–6.

Lightwood, R. (1956) The home care of sick children. *Practitioner*, **177**: 143.

MacFarlane, A. (1992) Personal child health record held parents. *Archives of Disease in Childhood*, **67**: 571–2.

Ministry of Health (1959). *The Welfare of Children in Hospital* (Platt Report). (London: HMSO).

Northway, W.H. (1990) Bronchopulmonary dysplasia: then and now. *Archives of Disease in Childhood*, **65**: 1076–81.

Ray, L. and Richie, J. (1993) Caring for chronically ill children at home: factors that influence parents coping. *Journal of Paediatric Nursing*, **8**: 4.

Robertson, J. and Robertson, J. (1989) *Separation and the Very Young*. (London: Free Association Books).

Royal College of Nursing (1993) *Buying Paediatric Community Nursing: A Guide for Purchasers and Commissioners of Health Care*. (London: RCN).

Royal College of Nursing (1995) *Directory of Paediatric Community Nursing Services*. (London: RCN).

Sainsbury, R., Hirst, M. and Lawton, D. (1995) *An Evaluation of Disability Living Allowance and Attendance Allowance*. Department of Social Security Research Report No. 41. (London, HMSO).

Smellie, J.M. (1956) Domicillary nursing service for infants and children. *British Medical Journal*, **5**: 256.

Southall, D.P. and Samuels, M.P. (1990) Bronchopulmonary dysplasia: a new look at management. *Archives of Disease in Childhood*, **65**: 1089–95.

Tatman, M.A. and Woodruffe, C. (1993) Paediatric home care in the UK. *Archives of Disease in Childhood*, **69**: 677–80.

Tatman, M.A., Woodruffe, C., Kelly, P.J. and Harris, R.J. (1992) Paediatric home care in Tower Hamlets: a working partnership with parents. *Quality in Health Care*, **1**: 98–103.

Thornes, R. (1993) *Bridging the Gaps. Caring for Children in the Health Services. An Exploratory Study of the Interface Between Primary and Specialist Care for Children Within the Health Services*. (London: Action for Sick Children).

While, A.E., Citrone, C. and Cornish, J. (1995) A study of the needs and provisions for families caring for children with life limiting incurable disorders. Unpublished report, Department of Health, London.

Whiting, M. (1988) Community paediatric nursing in England. MSc thesis, University of London.

Whiting, M., Goldman, L., and Manly, S. (1994) Meeting needs. Registered sick children's nurses in the community. *Paediatric Nursing*, **6**(1): 9–11.

Whyte, D.A. (1992) Family nursing approach to the care of a child with a chronic illness. *Journal of Advanced Nursing*, **17**: 317–27.

Further reading

Beresford, B. (1995) *Expert Opinions: A National Survey of Parents Caring for Disabled Children*. (London: Policy Press).

Jennings, P. (1994) Learning through experience: an evaluation of hospital at home. *Journal of Advanced Nursing*, **19**(5): 905–11.

12

CHILD PROTECTION IN PAEDIATRIC AMBULATORY CARE SETTINGS

Catherine Powell and Deborah Perriment

Child protection is the promotion of decisive action to prevent the maltreatment of children. While the majority of health-based child protection work takes place in community settings, nurses working in paediatric ambulatory care are likely to meet child protection issues in the course of their work. Nurses may need to develop their unique role in recognising and responding to cases of possible abuse and neglect. This work is both multidisciplinary and multiagency and involves working in partnership with the child and their family. Although there has been a tradition of limited support, advice and training in child protection available to paediatric nurses, this chapter provides an outline of the child protection framework and describes one model of practice, developed within an acute hospital trust, that is meeting the challenges of child protection and developing a possible way forward for good practice elsewhere.

Introduction

Child abuse and neglect is an important public health issue and represents a major, preventable cause of childhood morbidity and mortality. While all children should be considered to be vulnerable to the possibility of maltreatment, children who have health care problems related to physical or learning disabilities, a chronic illness or a pre-term birth may be particularly at risk (Westcott, 1993; Blumenthal, 1994). Such children and their families are likely to be frequent visitors to ambulatory care settings.

This chapter considers the unique role of the paediatric nurse in relation to child protection. Importantly, this role is seen to encompass a potential for preventative work as well as the early identification and referral of children who are at risk of, or suspected of suffering, abuse or neglect. While paediatric nurses in ambulatory care settings may provide care to children whose presenting health problems are a result of abuse, it is more likely that abuse or neglect (including sexual and emotional abuse) may be considered indirectly alongside other presenting health care problems.

Nurses working with children have developed the skills to challenge both medical and nursing practice. Models of working in partnership with children and their families are firmly established in many children's departments and hospitals. Much has been achieved in enhancing the quality of health care for children. Paediatric nurses need to be prepared to accept the challenge of their professional responsibilities in child protection. Through understanding this role, there will be a realisation that the task in child protection is too large and complex for any one individual practitioner or agency.

Good practice in child protection is facilitated by access to high-quality clinical supervision, training and support. The post of child protection nurse specialist working exclusively in an acute Trust, discussed later in the chapter, may be seen as an important innovation in working towards the protection of greater numbers of children from abuse and neglect.

Although this chapter is primarily written for nurses and other health care professionals working in ambulatory care settings (such as A&E departments, outpatients departments and day care areas), it is important to note that the major health care impetus in child protection lies with children's services in the community (Department of Health and Welsh Office, 1995). The health visitor's and school nurse's roles in child protection are particularly well established and well supported.

Success in child protection is dependent on interagency communication and collaboration. This will include liaison with community child health staff at the primary–secondary care interface. Nevertheless, the most important guiding principle, echoed in the Children Act 1989, is that, because of their age and vulnerability, the welfare of children is paramount.

Child protection

Child protection is the promotion of decisive action to protect children from abuse and neglect (Home Office et al., 1991). The importance of the concept of child protection (rather than non-accidental injury, for example) reflects the response to the recommendations of the public inquiries in to the deaths of children at the hands of their parents and carers. In particular, it was the death of 4½-year-old Jasmine Beckford and the subsequent inquiry (London Borough of Brent, 1985) that led to the publication of government guidelines aimed at improving interagency working in the field of child abuse and neglect (Department of Health and Social Security, 1988).

These first *Working Together* guidelines called for changes in professional practice among those working with at-risk children from a reactive to a proactive approach, the first duty of agencies caring for children being to protect the child from harm. The document provided clarity for action by workers in cases of actual or suspected child abuse. While the statutory agencies were identified as social services departments, the National Society for the Prevention of Cruelty to Children (NSPCC) and the police, the document also considered the roles of workers in health, education, probation and the voluntary sector.

The *Working Together* guidelines have since been updated in the light of the Children Act 1989. They continue to promote the importance of interagency communication and collaboration in child protection work. In particular, the guidelines highlight the *major role* that health care agencies have in protecting children from abuse and neglect, and participating in interagency work (Home Office *et al.*, 1991). This work may be complex and challenging. Dingwall *et al.* (1995) warn of the dangers inherent in taking an optimistic view that least stigmatises parents but may be lethal for the child.

The underlying philosophy of the legislation and guidance promotes children's rights as individuals and recognises the need to work in partnership with children and their families to ensure the best outcome for the child. Working in partnership with children and families is a key principle of effective paediatric nursing. However, there may be times when the notion of partnership with parents is challenged by the need to act in the best interest of the child. This is particularly so in the early stages of some child protection inquiries. Discussions with the multiagency team will most effectively establish the correct level of parental involvement. The recently published report into the prevention of child abuse found a clear link between greater parental involvement and better outcomes for the child (National Commission of Inquiry into the Prevention of Child Abuse, 1996).

Children's rights are linked to wider practice in child protection and may include issues of consent and restraint for medical investigations and treatment. In the UK, the recently published charter *The Patient's Charter: Services for Children and Young People* (Department of Health, 1996) celebrates many child- and family-centred innovations in paediatric care. Internationally, the United Nations Convention on the Rights of the Child 1989 promotes the need for legislation and social change to ensure that children have a life free from all forms of abuse, including negligent treatment and exploitation.

Defining abuse

Child abuse is not easily defined (or measured). One of the problems in child protection work is in defining a particular situation as child abuse. In addition, acts that may be constructed as abusive will vary across time and culture (Cloke and Naish, 1992; Rogers *et al.*, 1992). While the modern-day discovery of abuse is often attributed to the work of Kempe *et al.* (1962), who coined the term 'battered child syndrome' in relation to physical abuse, more recent attention has been given to other forms of abuse such as sexual abuse and emotional maltreatment. Although useful, the working definitions given in the official guidelines are not exclusive but categorise four different types of abuse – physical injury, neglect, sexual abuse and emotional abuse – for child protection registration purposes (Home Office *et al.*, 1991). These categories indicate a range of circumstances for which protective action is needed.

Recognition of child maltreatment

In paediatric ambulatory care, health professionals see a mere snapshot of a child and his relationships. The nature of care provision means that contact with the child and family will be brief and fragmented. Nevertheless, nurses in ambulatory care settings may be the first professionals to assess a child and note physical or behavioural indicators suggestive of possible abuse or neglect. These indicators are well documented elsewhere (see Hobbs *et al.*, 1993; Meadow, 1993; Blumenthal, 1994; Powell, 1995, for example), but in summary may include unusual bruising of soft tissue, burns, fractures, bite marks, failure to thrive, developmental delay, frozen watchfulness, sadness, self-mutilation, childhood overdose, indiscriminate attachment, precocious sexual activity, venereal disease and genital or rectal bleeding. The neglected child may present as unkempt, underweight and hungry.

Childhood abuse and neglect may contribute to both short-term and long-term health problems. Prognosis is likely to be less good where a family situation can be described as one of 'low warmth – high criticism' (Department of Health, 1995). These families may well be familiar to nurses working in ambulatory care settings. These families will be best served by early identification and referral of their problems coupled with extensive education and support in the experience of parenting. These interventions may help to reduce the risk to the children.

Protecting children with special needs presents particular difficulties. Such children may have communication problems, possess low self-esteem and be somewhat isolated. While such factors might contribute to additional vulnerability to abuse (Hobbs et al., 1993), they can also add to the difficulty of recognising that abuse has taken place. Furthermore, challenging behaviour, such as self-mutilation, may be more comfortably attributed to the child's intrinsic condition rather than the fact that abuse has occurred.

Children who also require special consideration are those from ethnic minorities. Here, professionals may be reluctant to be seen to implicitly criticise the cultural practices of others. Professionals may also believe that certain groups, for example those of Asian origin, are less likely to abuse. This may lead to a failure to protect children from harmful practices (Charles, 1993). Stereotyping of families also occurs within the dominant culture. An example of this may be a greater reluctance by professionals to interpret and acknowledge signs of abuse from within middle-class families.

The signs and symptoms of abuse are not definitive. They will always need to be taken in context with other factors. For nurses working in A&E departments, these factors may include concerns relating to the timescale in seeking help and a mismatch between the injuries and the explanations given. Concerns may also embrace the frequency of attendance in the department (Powell, 1997; Royal College of Nursing, 1997).

Child abuse is rarely a one-off incident, children who are seriously injured or killed often having a long history of frequent bruising and other injuries. In recognition of this factor, many A&E departments have information systems that highlight frequent attendees. It is also considered good practice to inform the child's general practitioner and health visitor or school nurse of the attendance. In tandem with this, it is important to have mechanisms in place that detect abusing parents and carers who shop around for health care in an attempt to conceal the repeated nature of their children's injuries or illness.

As significant as notifying attendance to A&E departments is communication of the fact that a child has failed to attend a clinic or department for investigations or treatment. The NCIPCA report recommends that all missed outpatients appointments are followed up (National Commission of Inquiry into the Prevention of Child Abuse, 1996). Acts of omission may be viewed as being as equally abusive as the more obvious non-accidental physical injury. A summary report of inquiries into the deaths of children from abuse and neglect (Department of Health, 1991) points to a characteristic period of silence prior to the death, whereby the child may have failed to receive the appropriate monitoring, support or health care. The parent-held child health record empowers the family in the ownership of information relating to children's health care needs. Professionals working in ambulatory care settings should help to ensure that the full potential of this document is realised.

Many centres offering paediatric ambulatory care will have an attached liaison health visitor. The key role of the postholder is to help to ensure two-way communication of concerns between primary and secondary care health professionals. The liaison health visitor will be reliant on the skills of paediatric nurses and others in the identification of children for whom there is a possible child protection concern.

Interestingly, Dingwall *et al.* (1995) comment that permanent nursing staff working in children's clinics and A&E departments often have detailed knowledge of the social geography of the local community. They suggest that this knowledge, alongside experience and skills in assessing parental demeanour, may be helpful in identifying possible abuse. Such skills are contrasted with the more limited attributes of junior doctors.

Implications for practice

The nurses' role in child protection in the UK lies within the framework of legislation and government guidelines for interagency working. As we have seen, this points to a proactive role in prevention, the early detection of family dysfunction and the provision of support. Cloke and Naish (1992) suggest that nurses have a role in prevention through the promotion of positive parenting and by working with parents to teach them normal patterns of development. Preventative work in child protection is correspondingly dependent upon the knowledge and understanding of a child's needs and rights as an individual. Such concepts are now enshrined in children's nursing practice.

The guidance document for senior nurses working in child protection, published in conjunction with the government guidelines, suggests that:

> Nurses, health visitors and midwives have a crucial part to play in protecting children. They may have regular contact and access not shared by other professionals. As a result, they will often be the first people able to identify children who need help or protection; and they may also be involved in enabling parental access to children.

> Therefore all nurses who come into contact with children must have a clear understanding of their duties and responsibilities, as well as their relationship with managers, other members of multi-disciplinary, multi-agency teams, and to those nurses with special responsibility for child protection. (Department of Health, 1997, p. 1)

In addition to understanding the child protection framework and being knowledgeable about indicators of possible abuse and neglect, nurses practising in ambulatory care settings will need to know how to respond to their suspicions that a child is being maltreated.

Responding

In most cases, the first step will be to discuss the nature of concerns with a senior nurse or doctor experienced in child protection. When a child presents with signs of possible abuse or neglect, it may also be useful to gather information from community staff such as health visitors, school nurses and general practitioners. The liaison health visitor may be able to give support in facilitating this.

The child should be referred to, and examined by, a paediatrician experienced in child protection. In some cases, it may be more appropriate for the child to be seen in a community clinic or health centre. Repeated examinations are to be avoided and may well be construed as further abuse by a child who is already traumatised. Social services departments, as the lead agency, may be able to offer advice and support at this early stage. A search of their records may show a previous concern within the family; in some cases, the child (or a sibling's) name may have previously been entered on the local child protection register. Many A&E departments have direct access to the names of children on the register. These children have already had a need for protection identified, and early communication with the key worker is imperative.

As a result of the medical examination and discussion of concerns with appropriate colleagues, a decision may be made to make a formal child protection referral to the local social services department. The precise mechanisms for achieving this will vary according to local guidelines and procedures. As the *Working Together* document (Home Office *et al.*, 1991) identifies, the responsibility for the provision of multiagency guidelines lies with the Area Child Protection Committee (ACPC). Individual agencies will usually have their own procedures that are commensurate with the ACPC guidelines. All nurses working with children should have access to, and be knowledgeable about, local guidelines, policies and procedures.

The process of protecting children will usually involve multidisciplinary assessment, followed as necessary by an interagency strategy discussion, social services investigation and a child protection conference. The child protection conference is a forum in which interagency professionals exchange information about the child and family. In recent times, it has been usual practice for the parents, and where appropriate the child, to be present and to contribute to the proceedings. At the conference, a decision will be made in respect of placing the child's name on to the child protection register under one or more of the categories of abuse (see above). Where this happens, a protection plan will be formulated and a social worker allocated to provide support and supervision as necessary. The case will then be reviewed (3–6 monthly) at further conferences and deregistration considered. It is important to note that the majority of children who are on the child protection register will remain in the care of their families (Department of Health, 1995). For some cases, criminal or care proceedings may follow. Because nurses may contribute at all stages of the child protection process, it is important that clear, contemporaneous records are kept.

Parents or carers will need to be supported and informed of any referral to a statutory agency. It is usual practice for parents to be fully involved in the assessment and investigation of possible abuse and neglect. However, there may be occasions when parents and carers present a threat to the child by removal from the clinic or department before treatment and investigations are completed. Under Section 46 of the Children Act (1989) 'police protection' allows the police to prevent removal of a child for up to 72 hours if they believe that a child would otherwise suffer significant harm.

Confidentiality

Child protection work involves working with other disciplines and agencies. In contrast to usual practice detailed in the Code of Professional Conduct, nurses may be required to share what is often very sensitive information with other parties. However, the key to protecting children is interagency communication and collaboration in the best interests of the child. Disclosure of information in relation to child protection by medical or nursing staff is considered a matter of public interest and will therefore normally be justified (Department of Health et al., 1994; UKCC, 1996).

The child protection nurse specialist

In England and Wales, each district health authority is required to identify a senior doctor, senior nurse (with a health visiting qualification) and senior midwife to take a lead in child protection. The so-called 'designated nurse' is usually a senior manager of community-based community nursing services. Designated nurses have increasingly devolved some of the responsibilities of child protection support and training to child protection nurse specialists, usually experienced health visitors. However, as the RCN (1994) found, the limited input to child protection in acute settings (including ambulatory care areas) by designated nurses and their deputies was further challenged by the creation of the market economy in health care and widespread generation of separate acute and community Trusts. So, although an increasing number of community staff had a remit for child protection responsibilities written into their job descriptions, there was the danger that hospital-based paediatric nurses' access to training and support would diminish.

Yet guidance on the clarification of the responsibilities of senior health professionals recommends that, in addition to the designated professionals, 'named professionals' (doctors and nurses/midwives) are available within each Trust. The duty of such professionals is to offer support and advice to staff concerned about child protection. The named professionals are also mandated to have a key role in the training, updating and clinical supervision of staff (Department of Health and Welsh Office, 1995). Thus where separate acute services and community Trusts have been established (as is the case in the authors' locality), there was an unique opportunity to secure on-site child protection support and training for staff working in ambulatory care settings.

The establishment of a child protection nurse specialist post in the authors' acute trust was an innovation that preceded both the government guidance and the RCN study (RCN 1994b; Department of Health and Welsh Office, 1995). The main activities of the post-holder include:

- the clinical supervision of staff involved in child protection cases (including advice and support, report-writing and supporting staff attending child protection conferences or court)
- the monitoring of cases of child protection across the Trust
- the development of child protection training for all staff disciplines
- the provision of expertise to the Trust in the development of child protection procedures
- the liaison with other health and social agencies (including feedback to staff as to outcomes)
- the development of practice through participation in local and national child protection working groups
- the research into the needs of staff working in the acute sector
- the dissemination of information about the role at national and international conferences.

Anecdotal evidence to date suggests that the post has been successful in improving awareness of child protection within the Trust. It has also led to an increase in the number of referrals of children to the statutory agencies. It is hoped that this in turn has improved the identification of children at risk of or suffering from child abuse and neglect.

In addition, it is surmised that there may have been an increase in preventative work through early identification of those families needing support. This is important and comes at a time when there is recognition of the need to refocus children's services and resources into the prevention of abuse through welfare provision, family support and self-help initiatives, rather than undertaking costly child protection investigations (Department of Health, 1995; NCIPCA, 1996). The support and empowerment of children and families is enshrined in the philosophy of paediatric nursing.

Education and training

While the child protection nurse specialist can provide some training and updating of child protection for staff, nurses working in paediatric ambulatory care settings should take the responsibility to ensure that they access all available opportunities to develop their child protection knowledge and understanding (Department of Health and Welsh Office, 1995; English National Board, 1995). Ideally, education and training programmes should have a multiagency focus to reflect the *Working Together* philosophy. Two educational programmes that have been developed jointly by the English National Board and the Council for the Education and Training of Social Workers provide an introductory and more in-depth opportunity for study. As with all child protection work, support should be made available for staff undertaking these and other training courses (Ireland and Powell, 1997).

Conclusion

Nurses working in paediatric ambulatory care settings have a unique and important role in protecting children. This includes preventative measures in the early identification of children and families in need of support. Failure to protect children from abuse and neglect has resulted in childhood deaths and disabilities. The need for continued therapeutic intervention as a result of abuse may be lifelong. The ability of nurses and others to prevent such tragedies is dependent upon access to good clinical supervision, training and support. The role of the child protection nurse specialist working exclusively in an acute Trust may provide a cost-effective solution and model for future practice.

Thus in summary:

1. Nurses working in paediatric ambulatory care settings have a unique role in child protection.
2. Child protection work is multiagency and multidisciplinary.
3. Good practice in child protection is facilitated by access to high-quality clinical supervision, training and support.
4. The post of child protection nurse specialist, working exclusively in an acute Trust, may be seen as an important innovation in the protection of children from abuse and neglect.
5. The major health care impetus in child protection lies with community child health staff, and the primary–secondary interface provides important opportunities for collaborative protective work.
6. The most important guiding principle in child protection is that the welfare of the child is paramount.

References

Blumenthal, I. (1994) *Child Abuse: A Handbook for Health Care Practitioners.* (London: Arnold).

Charles, M. (1993) Child protection conferences: maximising their potential, in Owen, H. and Pritchard, J. (eds) *Good Practice in Child Protection: A Manual for Professionals.* (London: Jessica Kingsley).

Cloke, C. and Naish, J. (eds) (1992) *Key Issues in Child Protection for Health Visitors and Nurses.* (Harlow: Longman).

Department of Health (1991) *Child Abuse: A Study of Inquiry Reports 1980–1989.* (London: HMSO).

Department of Health (1995) *Child Protection: Messages from Research.* (London: HMSO).

Department of Health (1996) *The Patient's Charter: Services for Children and Young People.* (London: Department of Health).

Department of Health (1997) *Child Protection: Guidance for Senior Nurses, Health Visitors and Midwives,* 3rd edn. (London: HMSO).

Department of Health, British Medical Association, Conference of the Medical Royal Colleges (1994) *Child Protection: Medical Responsibilities.* (London: Department of Health).

Department of Health and Social Security (1988) *Working Together: A Guide to Interagency Co-Operation for the Protection of Children from Abuse.* (London: HMSO).

Department of Health and Welsh Office (1995) *Child Protection: Clarification of Arrangements Between the NHS and Other Agencies*. (London: Department of Health).
Dingwall, R., Eeklaar, J. and Murray, T. (1995) *The Protection of Children*, 2nd edn. (Aldershot: Avebury).
English National Board (1995) *Child Protection Education*. (London: ENB).
Hobbs, C., Hanks, H. and Wynne, J. (1993) *Child Abuse and Neglect: A Clinicians Handbook*. (Edinburgh: Churchill Livingstone).
Home Office, Department of Health, Welsh Office *et al.* (1991) *Working Together Under the Children Act 1989: A Guide to Arrangements for Interagency Co-operation for the Protection of Children from Abuse*. (London: HMSO).
Ireland, L.M. and Powell, C. (1997) Working together: the development of an introductory course in child protection. *British Journal of Nursing*, 6(12): 686–90.
Kempe, C.H., Silverman, F.N., Steele, B.F. *et al.* (1962) The battered child syndrome. *Journal of the American Medical Association*, **181**: 17–24.
London Borough of Brent (1985) *A Child in Trust: The Report of the Panel of Inquiry into the Circumstances Surrounding the Death of Jasmine Beckford*. (London: Borough of Brent).
Meadow, R. (ed.) (1993) *ABC of Child Abuse*, 2nd edn. (London: BMJ Publishing Group).
National Commission of Inquiry into the Prevention of Child Abuse (1996) *Childhood Matters: The Report of the National Commission of Inquiry in to the Prevention of Child Abuse*. (London: Stationery Office).
Powell, C. (1995) Health problems of young children, in Campbell, S. and Glasper, E.A. (eds) *Whaley and Wong's Children's Nursing*. (London: Mosby).
Powell, C. (1997) Child protection in the accident and emergency department. *Accident and Emergency Nursing*, 5(2): 61–120.
Rogers, S., Hevey, D., Roche, J. and Ash, E. (1992) *Child Abuse and Neglect: Facing the Challenge*. (Milton Keynes: Open University).
Royal College of Nursing (1994) *Nursing and Child Protection: An RCN Survey*. (London: RCN).
Royal College of Nursing (1997) *Protecting Children*, 2nd edn. (London: RCN).
UKCC (1996) *Guidelines for Professional Practice*. (London: UKCC).
Westcott, H. (1993) *Abuse of Children and Adults with Disabilities*. (London: NSPCC).

Further reading

Cloke, C. and Naish, J. (eds.) (1992) *Key Issues in Child Protection for Health Visitors and Nurses*. (Harlow: Longman).
Meadow, R. (ed.) (1993) *ABC of Child Abuse*, 2nd edn. (London: BMJ Publishing Group).
Rogers, S., Hevey, D., Roche, J. and Ash, E. (1992) *Child Abuse and Neglect: Facing the Challenge*. (Milton Keynes: Open University).
Royal College of Nursing (1997) *Protecting Children*, 2nd edn. (London: RCN).

13

CULTURE AND THE CHILD HEALTH AMBULATORY SETTING

Jim Richardson

Defining culture

Culture is an elusive term that means different things to different people. At first glance, culture may seem to be a very abstract issue, particularly when some of the definitions for culture derived from sociology and anthropology are considered. In fact, culture is a vital, everyday concept that is of the first importance for health care professionals and the people using their services. Articles dealing with culture in health care often start by emphasising that Britain is now a multicultural society (Weller, 1994), so that culture requires our attention if we are to provide an effective and respectful service for those to whom we offer care. This is clearly true (Skellington and Morris, 1992; Mason, 1995) but is only part of the story. Ethnic origin is one aspect of culture about which we readily become aware when working with children and families. As a highly visible aspect of culture, it is a topic about which considerable amounts of demographic information have been collected (Skellington and Morris, 1992; Balarajan and Raleigh, 1993). The sheer mass of information about just one facet of culture underscores the importance of this topic to health care workers.

Careful consideration of what culture is will reveal that culture in fact concerns everyone: adult, child, nurse, patient/client. Many people have tried to define what culture is (for example, Mashaba, 1995). In the popular mind, culture is often considered to be the high culture of artistic and creative work; a cultured person may be one who enjoys opera, ballet, classical literature or modern art. A growing awareness that the UK is the home of people of a range of national and ethnic origins has resulted in 'culture' being used to describe the differentness of these new Britons. This aspect can be seen in health care where culture is often called into question when the patient/client looks or sounds different from what is expected. This has led to early attempts to develop transcultural nursing, resulting in a focus on the 'exotic' and 'unusual'. At the same time, there has been a tendency to try to learn lists of facts about groups in society that are tangibly different. This has led to nurses making assumptions such as, 'This family is Sikh so they do A, B and C and not D, E and F.' This rather mechanistic approach is understandable in the face of a new situation requiring a new knowledge base and new skills. It may even be praiseworthy as an indication of a raised awareness of and sensitivity to the needs of the Sikh family, but it is a rather risky approach as it also implies a range of assumptions and stereotypes that may or may not be true of that particular Sikh family. Clearly, a more *versatile*, *flexible* approach will be required, which will inevitably involve asking the family involved to clarify issues.

It is possible to list the principal features of culture:

- *It is learned* – children learn their culture within their family and later at school and from peers. It follows that, as children learn their culture, there will be periods when the child's concept of culture is incomplete and particularly sensitive to the criticism or disrespect of others.
- *It is passed from generation to generation.*
- *It is dynamic* – it will change in transmission between generations and in response to the place and conditions in which those sharing the culture live.
- *It helps us to identify the group to which we 'belong'* and, by implication, the groups to which we do not belong.
- *It defines our core beliefs* – this will include religious belief. This may be extremely important to the family, particularly in time of crisis such as when a child is ill. It is all too easy to fail to display respect for someone else's religious beliefs, particularly when they differ from our own.
- *It defines our core values* – it helps us to judge 'right' and 'wrong'.
- *It influences our life habits and customs* – how we dress or the food that we eat are defined by culture, and we may be unwilling to accept anything which differs from these familiar patterns (Fieldhouse, 1995).
- *It gives us patterns for living* – it may guide how we respond to crises and life's difficulties generally (Danielson *et al.*, 1993).

- *It is important to us* – we are ready to assume that our ways are 'right' and to defend them against others. This explains why cultural questions can become the source of human conflict.
- *It is thoroughly internalised* – since we have learned about our culture from earliest childhood, it may be so much part of us as to be largely subconscious. We do not think of our cultural orientation in a conscious manner every time we are called upon to make for example an ethical judgement: it seems to come from the 'gut' level

This may make it seem that culture is a highly uniform phenomenon for those sharing it. A moment's thought, however, will reveal that individuals will naturally vary to some extent in the degree to which they accept, reject or live by the precepts of their culture. Everyone's life experience will lead to variations in this. This is important because we cannot assume that people conform to stereotypes. It is one of the important principles of transcultural nursing that: *if we want to know about someone's culture, we must ask them!*

After carefully considering these features of culture, it will become clear that culture is not simply an issue of nationality or race. In fact, culture is a much wider concept. It could be said that many different groups in society have a shared culture. On this basis, we could say that different social classes or professional groups have a distinct culture, as may age groups such as adolescents or the elderly. Who would deny that people with different regional origins, such as the Welsh, Yorkshire people or those from the Black Country, have distinctive cultures? It could be argued that the genders have distinctive cultures. In fact, whenever children's nurses experience difficulties working with a client family, culture should be suspected as a probable cause.

One of the major aims of transcultural nursing is to lead nurses to consider the role that their own culture plays in relationships with those to whom they offer care. It is easy for us to assume that our cultural orientation is correct and therefore unthinkingly to condemn the orientation of others as incorrect. Such ethnocentrism is a feature of all of us and can be very damaging in our relationships with others if we do not improve our self-awareness of the degree to which we allow it to influence our thinking and decisions. If we find ourselves working with people whose culture influences them to act in a way we do not expect, we can find ourselves suffering from culture shock. This can seriously compromise our ability to think, communicate and work with others. The potential effect of this phenomenon on those who visit ambulatory care facilities should be considered.

Ambulatory care

For the purposes of this chapter, ambulatory care will be defined in the broadest terms. This may include the care offered to children and their families in outpatients departments and A&E units, as ward attendees for follow-up after an episode of care in an acute area of a hospital, and in day surgical units and primary health care institutional care areas such as the child health clinic. Characteristic of all of these settings is the fact that the child comes to the health care professional and the duration of the contact is short (Stower, 1993), usually less than 24 hours. In this context, health promotion and prevention are obviously of prime importance. The family will return home to continue caring for the child so that the aim will be, after a short contact, to prepare the family with the knowledge and skills necessary to both undertake the child's basic care, and also to meet the demands of any enhanced health needs the child may have.

To achieve an effective interaction between the children's nurse and the child and family in an ambulatory setting, a systematic approach to the issues must be adopted. The process of nursing offers just such a framework, but central to the success of any approach must be the quality of communication and interaction between the child, family and nurse. Owing to the briefness of the encounter, it is of the utmost importance that clarity of communication and mutual understanding are achieved. There is little opportunity for the immediate recap of new material. However, the child and family may be required to act on this material as soon as they return home without having immediate recourse to the nurse to check on details. Culture is acknowledged as an issue that may act as an impediment to effective communication. This chapter will focus on the role of an understanding of cultural issues in ensuring clear, effective communication and collaboration between children's nurses and children and their families in an ambulatory care setting.

Culture and communication

There are many points at which culture can act as a stumbling block between children's nurses and their patients/clients who are trying to understand each other. There may be the obvious communication difficulty if the nurse and client family do not speak the same language. A range of communication strategies can be used to overcome this gulf (Slater, 1993). Many ambulant care facilities make use of interpreters and link workers from the communities using that facility. Of course, if this is to be a successful strategy, there are a number of basic rules to be observed:

1. The interpreter or link worker must be properly prepared for this task:
   - It is clearly unsatisfactory if the interpreter 'chooses' what to translate and leaves untranslated what he or she feels is not significant.
   - The translator must have a command of the professional jargon used in the health care setting.
   - The translator must understand and be committed to maintaining professional ethical standards, for example confidentiality.
2. The interpreter must be socially acceptable to the target community:
   - It may not be satisfactory to some communities for a young, unmarried female interpreter to attempt to enquire about the obstetric history of a sick child's mother. It may be felt that she should not know about such things as a single woman.
   - For some communities, the match between the social class of the client family and that of the interpreter must be considered. Families might well be reluctant to reveal personal information to someone who is considered to be of a different social class with whom the family would normally have no social contact.
3. The use of informal interpreters should be avoided:
   - It may tempting to ask one of the family's older children to interpret. In some communities, the female members of the family may have minimal contact with the majority culture and thus have little opportunity to learn English. The family's children, however, generally learn the language quickly at school. This may make them seem like the ideal interpreter. This must, however, be avoided as it may alarm and embarrass everyone involved.
   - In the same way, male relatives may seem like a good option as interpreters. Men, through work, often have more opportunity to learn English. This situation would require an under-

standing of gender roles in the family's culture and what may or may not be 'decently' spoken of.

- Some health care facilities keep a list of employees who can interpret in an emergency. This may be useful in gathering basic information. However, the employee may not be well versed in health issues: the kitchen porter cannot be expected to interpret information on signs, symptoms and health history, and may be of a different community or social class from the patient's family.
- Informal interpreters cannot be expected to understand the ethical requirements of their task.

Written communication is another area in which cultural issues are important. In the ambulant care setting, this will be especially significant since written communication in the form of information sheets and so on is often provided for the family to take home with them after the care episode. Consideration must be given to a number of factors:

- If leaflets and other forms of information provided are in English, is the level of language used appropriate? Official agencies have often been criticised for providing information in a written format appropriate to the writer, for example at the level of an educated professional. Not everyone has the advantage of this level of education.
- What provision is made for the parent and/or child who is not literate? This is an issue for the family whose members have never learned to read or who learned to read another language. Excellent progress has been made in ensuring the provision of information leaflets in a range of languages, such as those spoken in India, Pakistan and Bangladesh. These are, however, useless if the speaker of one of these languages happens to be illiterate. More creative means to communicate information, such as audiocassettes or videos, should be investigated.
- Are written materials attractively produced? It requires some motivation to plough through an information sheet, and the recipient may be reluctant to invest this sort of effort if the leaflet is awkwardly laid out, poorly written and badly photocopied.

Of course, there is always a potential for misunderstanding when the nurse speaks with a child and family who share her language. Factors such as regional dialect, social class differences in speech and professional jargon can all compromise mutual understanding. Equally, the children's nurse must take the child's cognitive ability and experience into account when attempting to communicate purposefully with that child (Richardson, 1996).

The children's nurse must also preserve an awareness of non-verbal communication issues. The use of gestures can be interpreted differently in different cultures. Gaze can be employed to communicate different things in different cultural groups; some use it to convey closeness and sincerity, while others may use it as a challenge. For some groups, sustained eye contact may convey social superiority and might imply disrespect; such groups may particularly emphasise that children should avoid engaging eye contact with adults in order to convey respect for their elders.

When communicating, the children's nurse must bear in mind different cultures' interpretation of the use of social space (Giger and Davidhizar, 1991). In some cultures, it is necessary for those communicating to be in close proximity; if arm's length distance, such as is comfortable for British people, is maintained, this may be felt to transmit coolness and a lack of care. On the other hand, if the nurse stands very close to someone from a culture that emphasises the need for a generous social space, this might be felt to be intrusive and disrespectful. This issue is one which is familiar to children's nurses since children are generally sensitive to physical proximity and the nurse is well used to interpreting the ideal distance when communicating by interpreting the child's reaction.

Time is an issue that has a bearing on communication (Boyle and Andrews, 1989). Some cultures, such as the UK majority culture, value highly what they see as the efficient use of time. For these cultures, time is a valued commodity: 'Time is money.' Such people may feel that punctuality is very important and that social interactions should be brief and to the point. From this point of view, it may be easy to condemn other cultures' failure to ascribe to this point of view. Many cultures adopt a much more leisurely approach to time-keeping and may not share the British sense of urgency in reliably being on time. This may be illustrated when some families seem to be unaware of the importance we attach to being on time for events such as appointments at ambulatory care facilities. It is all too easy for the children's nurse to *misinterpret* this attitude as a casual disregard for the facilities offered by the health service (Waddell and Peterson, 1994). To underscore that this is not simply an issue in dealing with those whose national origins are outside the UK, it should be remembered that a sense of the importance of precise time-keeping may become less important to people who have been long-term unemployed. Another aspect of the same issue is that some cultural orientations will lead people to expect that the children's nurse will devote a good deal of time to communicating with them, while others will assume that the nurse is a busy, efficient professional who will devote only enough time to them to communicate the essential information and answer their immediate questions. Deciding how best to achieve mutual understanding in the optimal use of time is another question of interpretation.

Another factor related to cultural attitudes to time is the family's time orientation (Richardson, 1994). The family may be past, present or future orientated. With a past orientation, tradition in dealing with illness or other difficulties may be emphasised. If the family tends to be present orientated, they may be solely concerned with the here-and-now and find it difficult to share health care professionals' concern for current action for future health improvement. For the children's nurse, who, in our society, is generally future orientated, it is natural to anticipate that present sacrifices, in the form of the investment of time and energy, might be expected of the client family. A concrete example of this may be seen in compliance with long-term drug therapy for a disease such as tuberculosis. The nurse understands that this disorder requires antibiotic treatment for 6–12 months to eradicate it completely. The family, however, may have difficulty in putting up with the effort this may require, particularly if the child looks and feels well a short time after starting the treatment.

Another very important cultural issue in communication concerns to whom communication is addressed. Children's nurses in the UK are accustomed to addressing children directly in acknowledgement of their right to be treated as unique individuals. Our society also treats mothers as being of primary importance in children's health and welfare. However, we must take into account *who* in the family may expect to be addressed. As I have previously outlined, the traditional division of responsibilities in family life characteristic of some cultural groups requires that the father be accorded the respect of having communication focus on him. The mother and child may modestly reject direct questions from a stranger outside the family and instead defer to the father. Another feature of the same phenomenon is that the family may be taken aback by being offered information and instructions from a young, female children's nurse. Whenever communication appears not to be flowing smoothly, it is worthwhile pausing for a moment to consider whether these issues might be at the root of the difficulty. It is neither sensible nor useful to feel insulted if confronted by problems such as these. The client family will be showing their lack of insight into the mechanics of the social roles and interaction in the majority culture, just as the nurse might initially lack insight into their conventions for social behaviour. As in all intercultural interactions, the solution lies in negotiation. Careful assessment of the family's responses will indicate whether there is a problem and what questions need to be asked in order to resolve that problem.

CASE STUDY 1

K., a 7-year-old boy, requires outpatient treatment for his psoriasis. His family are travelling people with their roots in Ireland. There has been great difficulty in organising consistent care for K. as his family move frequently. This has been partially solved by K.'s family holding his medical records, which they present whenever they seek treatment for K.'s skin complaint. At this point, K.'s psoriasis is so severe that it is felt that he needs drug treatment. This treatment is well established but has potentially dangerous side-effects. This is explained to K. and his mother, but they seem reluctant to consider this treatment. Rather than accept the family's apparent rejection of the treatment, the children's nurse chats further with them about their reluctance to discuss the treatment on offer. K.'s mother explains in response that she does not want to make a decision alone on such an important question. She reveals that, to consider the issue further, she would like to talk to her grandmother. In her culture, the elder women in the family are highly regarded for their wisdom and wide experience of life. Another outpatients appointment is arranged, which K.'s great-grandmother can attend so she can participate in the discussion of K.'s treatment options.

As a professional carer, the children's nurse has a range of knowledge and skills in the field of child health and illness. Such knowledge and skills are generally rooted in a Western scientific biomedical philosophy of health and disease. This may form the first barrier to mutual understanding as the client family may explain health and illness in quite a different manner (Stainton Rogers, 1991; Helman, 1994).

CASE STUDY 2

Mr J., an unemployed man previously employed in a traditional industry, is now occupied in caring for his children at home while his wife works in a recently opened electronics factory in their home town in industrial South Wales. He brings his 4-year-old daughter to a drop-in clinic at the paediatric unit of the local district general hospital. He explains that he is worried that his daughter is about to become seriously ill, but his GP does not appear to take his concerns seriously. The basis of his worry is that his daughter has twice recently had head lice. It would be very easy for the nurse to dismiss this concern because she knows that head lice are a common but minor health issue in childhood. However, the nurse who understands the health beliefs of people living in this area would know that there are still vestiges of an old belief that all children have the potential to have head lice but that these only appear when the child is debilitated and about to become very ill. Mr J. may be disadvantaged because he may not be able to explain his concern clearly. As a house-husband, he is occupying a new role, for which his upbringing has not prepared him. He may feel uncomfortable doing what he considers to be 'women's work' and feel unprepared to answer the health care profes-sionals' questions. Mr J. may suspect the nurses' and doctors' expertise if he is simply offered malathion shampoo to treat his daughter's lice. This may indicate to him that they do not 'know' how serious his daughter's health problem is and are not offering treatment for the apparently underlying problem.

In talking with people from different cultural backgrounds, it is important to consider how we communicate respect. One device is the way in which we address people. A grandparent who brings a child to the clinic may naturally be taken aback to be referred to as 'Gran' as the older generation place perhaps more emphasis on the use of formal titles, such as Mr or Mrs plus surname, than do today's young parents. It also conveys an attitude of casual disre-spect if we get people's names wrong. There is, of course, great potential for mistakes when the family's name is very different from the British norm and family members do not necessarily share a surname (Schott and Henley, 1996). With a little effort, each indi-vidual's full name can be clarified and recorded. This information is also significant because mistakes may lead to the child's nursing and medical records being misfiled and effectively lost.

Many formats for cultural assessment in nursing have been proposed (for example, Dobson, 1991), but these tend to be complex and ill suited for rapid, everyday use. The nurse specialising in transcultural issues may well use these, but the generalist children's nurse is unlikely to find them practical or helpful. Perhaps the most important thing the generalist nurse can do in the majority of client interactions is to maintain a *sensitivity* to cultural issues. This will ensure that the appropriate information is sought using the assessment method employed in that particular clinic or unit. Activities of daily living can be investigated with a cultural slant to ensure that the appropriate questions are asked of the child and family. In particularly difficult situations, it will be important to appreciate when someone with more expertise in this area should be consulted.

Culture and families

The family as an idea is striking in its diversity (Benokraitis, 1993). We often think of the family as a mother, father and 2.3 children, which is the most common variant in our society. However, variability is seen in the increasingly common variants of family, such as the single-parent family and the blended family resulting from divorce and remarriage. These norms are strongly influenced by culture and are dynamic in the same way that culture is dynamic. A generation ago, it would have been unthinkable that two lesbians or gay men would form stable emotional and economic unions that would form a family in which children could be cared for and raised. The form of family that is prevalent is affected by many factors, for example the economic climate. We have seen geographical mobility become a much more common phenomenon as people move to different parts of the country to seek work and advancement. This often has the effect that the extended family structure is ruptured by physical distance. Older relatives who might have offered considerable support and assistance are left behind while same-generation friends and colleagues in the location take on a greater significance in providing such practical help. This will, of course, also be the effect experienced by families who have relocated by immigration.

Roles within families are also subject to the same evolution. In the UK, there has been change in the traditional mother's and father's role as more women exercise their right to continue their careers after having children. Many cultures are rather less tolerant of this sort of innovation and strongly emphasise the importance of the female role within the household. This may extend to the maintenance of traditional 'spheres of responsibility' within the family, which will dictate who decides on issues affecting the family. In some societies, the eldest male will be expected to make decisions with regard to the family's contact with the outside world, while the female will be decisive in choices relating to the family's well-being within the home. In practical terms, this can lead to a degree of misunderstanding within the health care system, as is illustrated in Case Study 3.

CASE STUDY 3

Mrs S. comes to the paediatric ENT outpatient department with her 3-year-old daughter, R. R. has had recurrent ear infections, and audiometry has demonstrated that she has a degree of hearing loss. It is planned that R., who was on an earlier clinic visit highly resistant to being examined, should have an examination under sedation. The clinic staff ask Mrs S. for written consent to this procedure but she refuses, saying that she cannot give consent – only her husband can do this but he is at work. The clinic staff get quite exasperated at this situation, saying that she is the child's mother and an adult so should be able to consent to treatment. Mrs S. finds the clinic staff's attitude quite threatening and hurtful and is inclined to leave before R. can be examined.

This situation arises from a mutual lack of understanding. If the clinic staff were culturally sensitive, they would appreciate the importance of this division of labour in decision-making, either emphasising the importance of R.'s father coming to the clinic, trying to call him to the clinic or making a later appointment that Mr S. could attend with his wife and daughter. It is not necessary for nurses to have knowledge of the customs of every cultural group with regard to this sort of situation, but it is important that they have an awareness that decision-making and consent is an area where there may be some variation – and that they plan to accommodate such difference.

The family can be seen as the cradle of culture. It is within the family that the norms, values, customs and beliefs of the wider society in general and the family group in particular are consolidated and transmitted to new generations. Children receive instruction on what is 'right' and 'wrong' and watch their parents, older siblings and others in the kin group as role models. This can often be seen in play, where children act out their observations on, for example, how the sexes interact in games of Mummies and Daddies. Children can see the formalities of social relationships between adults and can copy these. At the same time, the behaviour expected of children is outlined and enforced. Many cultures expect a high degree of deference from children in their dealings with adults. In some languages, it is expected that the child use respectful forms of speech, such as 'vous' in French rather than the informal 'tu', which may, in turn, be used by an adult talking to a child.

Standards of behaviour are defined through the discipline expected in the home and through formal and informal instruction. Formal instruction may be through the medium of, for example, religious education, while informal instruction may be communicated through more subtle cues. In many cultures, children's exploration of their own bodies and masturbation are viewed with discomfort by adults. This rarely takes the form of discussion but is nevertheless effectively communicated to children through disapproval and avoidance of directly addressing the issue.

Conclusion

Culture is an issue that is central to *all* of us but is so much part of us that we may not always consider it as a factor in our dealings with others. Nevertheless, culture plays a vital role in defining our behaviour, reactions to others and communication with them. Without a degree of self-awareness concerning culture, it can be a damaging and impeding factor preventing us from achieving mutual understanding and satisfying and constructive collaboration.

Culture will be a component of every interaction between children's nurses and the children and their families who use the health services. If we take this issue into account, we improve the chances that our therapeutic, professional relationships can be based on mutual understanding and take into account the *whole* child and *whole* family. Culture should be recognised as the ordinary, everyday phenomenon it is rather than just an exotic and unusual idea.

References

Balarajan, R. and Raleigh, V.S. (1993) *Ethnicity and Health: A Guide for the NHS.* (London: Department of Health).

Benokraitis, N.V. (1993) *Marriages and Families*. (Englewood Cliffs, New Jersey: Prentice-Hall).

Boyle, J.S. and Andrews, M.M. (1989) *Transcultural Concepts in Nursing Care*. (London: Scott, Foresman).

Danielson, C.B., Hamel-Bissell, B. and Winstead-Fry, P. (1993) *Families, Health and Illness: Perspectives on Coping and Intervention*. (London: Mosby).

Dobson, S.M. (1991) *Transcultural Nursing*. (London: Scutari Press).

Fieldhouse, P. (1995) *Food and Nutrition: Customs and Culture*, 2nd edn. (London: Chapman & Hall).

Giger, J.N. and Davidhizar, R.E. (1991) *Transcultural Nursing: Assessment and Intervention*. (London: Mosby Year Book).

Helman, C.G. (1994) *Culture, Health and Illness*, 3rd edn. (Oxford: Butterworth Heinemann).

Mashaba, G. (1995) Culture, in French, P. (ed.) *The Nurse, Self and Society: An Introduction to Applied Behavioural Sciences for Nurses and Health Care Professionals*. (Hong Kong: Waverly Info-Med).

Mason, S. (1995) *Race and Ethnicity in Modern Britain*. (Oxford: Oxford University Press).

Richardson, J. (1994) Cultural issues in critical care nursing, in Millar, B. and Burnard, P. (eds) *Critical Care Nursing*. (London: Baillière Tindall).

Richardson, J. (1996) Counselling children, in Burnard, P. and Hulatt, I. (eds) *Nurses Counselling: The View from the Practitioners*. (Oxford: Butterworth Heinemann).

Rogers, W. Stainton (1991) *Explaining Health and Illness: An Exploration of Diversity*. (London: Harvester Wheatsheaf).

Schott, J. and Henley, A. (1996) *Culture, Religion and Childbearing in a Multiracial Society*. (Oxford: Butterworth Heinemann).

Skellington, R. and Morris, P. (1992) *'Race' in Britain Today*. (London: Sage).

Slater, M. (1993) *Health for All Our Children: Achieving Appropriate Health Care for Black and Minority Ethnic Children and their Families*. (London: Action for Sick Children).

Stower, S. (1993) Innovative practice in the outpatient setting, in Glasper, E.A. and Tucker, A. (eds) *Advances in Child Health Nursing*. (London: Scutari Press).

Waddell, C. and Peterson, A.R. (1994) *Just Health: Inequality in Illness, Care and Prevention*. (Melbourne: Churchill Livingstone).

Weller, B. (1994) Cultural aspects of children's health and illness, in Lindsay, B. (ed.) *The Child and Family: Contemporary Nursing Issues in Child Health and Care*. (London: Baillière Tindall).

14

COMMUNITY OUTREACH FOR CHILDREN WITH COMPLEX NEEDS

Rachel E. Bia

This chapter draws upon the experience of setting up an Outreach Service for children with complex needs to illustrate the key aspects needed in community-based services to meet the needs of those who use them.

Such services have developed with the trend over the past decade for the community-based provision of care in response to government legislation and changing family support needs. Russell (1995) discusses the need for formal community-based networks, which have become necessary because of the major changes in family life, that is, increased family mobility, poverty, homelessness and single parenting. The extended family's role has diminished in many ways, requiring the need for community-based/home-based support, especially with very young children with complex needs where residential short-term care has been deemed inappropriate. The Children Act 1989 and *The Patient's Charter: Services for Children and Young People* (1996) in the UK have had a major influence on how services are provided to children with disabilities and, in the health service provision, on the emergence of paediatric community home care teams.

The development of the Outreach Service by The Children's Trust, Tadworth, has been in line with these changes of service delivery for children in general resulting from legislation and developments in paediatric nursing home care services.

Tatman and Woodroffe's survey in 1993 of specialist and general paediatric home care services concluded that, at that time, there were more specialist services (124) than general services (62), and that specialist paediatric home care teams were usually attached to a regional centre or hospital with specific expertise.

The similarity with other specialist services has been that the Outreach Service has developed from a specialist centre for children with complex needs. The Tadworth service can concur with Tatman and Woodroffe's findings that most paediatric home care services, whether general or specialist provision, are patchy but are growing rapidly across the UK.

There are many models of paediatric home care, as described by Peter and Torr (1996), Hughes (1997) and Gallagher (1996). All outline the setting-up of such services and their growth within existing UK NHS Trusts. The fundamental difference of the Tadworth Outreach Service is that it is a service that has emerged from an independent charity specialising in the care of children with complex needs. The aim of the service has been to provide specialised care by releasing the expertise of the Trust's staff to support parents and community professionals in the child's local area. The service works with and alongside local services, meeting the demand for a specialised nursing service where there is a lack of resources or gaps in service, predominantly in the south-east of England.

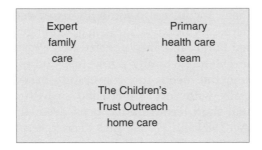

Figure 14.1 Partnership model for the Outreach Service
(adapted from Gould, 1996)

The need for liaison with the child's local community professionals has been paramount in order to inform local teams of the role of the Outreach Service and to avoid duplication and confusion. The Outreach Service has developed a partnership model adapted from Gould (1996) (Figure 14.1), whereby the family are seen as providing expert care with the support of the primary health care team and The Children's Trust Outreach home care. Casey *et al.* (1997) have discussed the implications of integrated services for children and have defined families' problem areas high-lighted by the Health Select Committee as:

- lack of co-ordination
- poor communication
- lack of specific education/training.

Kelly and colleagues (1994) suggest that promoting good experiences for families, better co-ordination of services and efficiency of service delivery are key aspects of a community service.

To illustrate the role of the Outreach Service, case studies will be used to describe the service model that was developed to address the balance between the care needs of the children and the training and support needs of Outreach staff. Through the staff working in partnership with the children's parents, there is a match between service provision and the child's and/or family's needs, as opposed to matching needs to a prescribed service. This fulfils one of the key requirements of *Caring for People: Community Care in the Next Decade and Beyond*, published by the UK government in 1989.

The idea of a Trust Outreach Service had long been considered but began to take shape in 1993, after a research study commissioned by The Children's Trust was conducted by The Norah Fry Institute (1993). This focused on future development possibilities for the Trust. One of the areas suggested was a home-based care service to provide the skills and expertise of the Trust's staff to children with complex needs. A survey of families already using the residential respite services was also conducted to ascertain the parents' views of this possible development. A questionnaire was sent out to families asking whether they would use such a service and on what basis, for example weekends, school holidays or nights. The response was very positive, leading to an application for Department of Health funding (from the Pilot Project funding for the development of services for children with life-threatening and life-limiting conditions (Department of Health, 1992). Two years' funding was granted to develop the service.

	Perceived and expressed need for Outreach Service	
Families Children	Development of service	Staff
Meet with parents to discuss their views of services required	Ascertain present availability of services and gaps in provision Ascertain regulations	Arrange information session Gain staff views
	Meet key personnel in health authorities and local authorities programmes	Set standards for staff Plan orientation, training and update sessions/
Gradually provide a service to children and families	Write a business plan Set service charges Draw up terms and conditions Produce leaflets Market the service Set standards for the service Construct audit tools Gain registration	Introduce existing and new staff to the service Build up team in response to demand for service Supervise, train, appraise and update on continuous basis

Evaluation of Service
by parents, staff and Outreach

Team to discuss current
service and identify areas of
improvement and future
development

Figure 14.2 Strategy for the development of an Outreach Service

The Outreach liaison nurse (later to become Outreach manager) was appointed in late 1994, charged with the brief of developing a strategy for the development of the service (Figure 14.2). This entailed ascertaining the present service availability, identifying gaps in provision and discussing with parents their views of how the service should develop. To function as a domiciliary service, the Outreach Service required under the Nursing Agencies Act 1959 the inspection and licence to function as a nursing agency and became a member of the United Kingdom Home Care Association (UKHCA) (1994), a major home care organisation that sets standards for home care providers. The Tadworth service is now one of the only few home care providers for children to function as a nursing/care agency and a member of the association in the UK. At the same time, information sessions were held with Trust staff to discuss the proposed service and the implications of service delivery into the community by the Trust. Staff who were interested in providing home-based care were identified, and the service gradually began with provision to children already known to the Trust. The new scheme soon gained recognition, and the demand for the service quickly outstripped the already limited services available. Referrals came from social workers, health authority purchasers and parents whose children had never used the Trust's services before but required the skills and expertise of the staff. Initially, the Outreach liaison nurse provided 'hands-on' care alongside developing the service during the first year, gradually building up a 'bank' of chil dren's learning disability and general trained nurses and care assistants. Some of these staff were from the established residential services, others were former Trust staff and some were new staff recruited specifically for the Outreach Service.

As the service demand grew, there was a need to employ staff in the areas of demand to provide a local, flexible service to the families. This required appropriately skilled staff or recruiting care staff who had the enthusiasm and commitment to work with children with complex needs. With the growth of staff numbers, the need for induction and ongoing training required a formalised system with the Outreach liaison nurse and Outreach nurse co-ordinator organising Saturday morning workshops (Saturday morning being the time when most staff could attend as most Outreach bank staff had other main employment during the week). The training/orientation of staff covered basics of care – safety in the home, resuscitation, the lifting and positioning of children, and confidentiality. The staff were then supported with supervision, and for care assistants the first session of providing care to a child was directly supported by the Outreach liaison nurse or nurse co-ordinator.

The Service has also formalised some principal standards:

1. No member of staff will be expected to provide care to a child/family until they have been formally introduced and/or supported through their first visit.

2. Each family and member of staff will be visited or seen at minimum on a monthly basis to assess the service satisfaction for the family and provide supervision for the staff.
3. Each child will have a qualified link nurse, who will co-ordinate the assessment, planning, implementation and evaluation of the service with the child, parents and staff involved.

The standards have arisen from the children's and parents' experiences of other services and the staff's identified needs for support and training. Parents do not want someone turning up on their doorstep who is neither prepared nor knowledgeable about their child's needs. The posts of Outreach liaison nurse and Outreach nurse co-ordinator have enabled staff (especially new staff) to be formally introduced and orientated to the specific child's needs in order to avoid, as one parent stated:

> every time we have someone new… I have to teach them, which really defeats the object of me having a carer come to the home.

Or, as another parent stated:

> The service we used in the past could only come at a certain time and would only provide someone if we went out… they would not feed or bath either.

Referrals have also come from within the Trust for children requiring home-based care and support as part of their planned discharge back to their local area, and from parents who wish to continue using short-term residential care but need a more flexible care package enabling a choice of where their child is cared for. Robinson (1995) has concluded, researched and written extensively about children with disabilities and their families' need for a choice of respite options, the need sometimes to have a complete break with residential respite, but also the option for their child to be cared for at home. Other referrals have been for children and families who have not used the Trust's facilities before but for whom, because of the child's complex needs or a lack of resources in the child's local area, Outreach was requested to provide a service. The referrals have often been seen as a last resort for many families because other services have not been able to provide the families with the support they need. Hubert (1991) believes that families with disabled children who have difficult behaviour to manage, incontinence or feeding difficulties are more likely to be families who have received little or no support. The referrals for the Outreach Service to be involved with children with complex needs and their families have included a 7-night-a-week service at home, supporting children with physical disabilities in mainstream schools and providing care and stimulation for children in their own homes during school holidays. To provide a flexible and responsive service, the Outreach Service has needed to employ nurses of all specialities, that is, Registered Children's Nurses, Registered Nurses (Learning Disabilities) and Registered General Nurses, especially when providing care to a wide range of children with disabilities. These staff may be, for example, children's nurses to provide services to highly dependent children who are continuously ventilated and, in the case of children with difficult or challenging behaviour, learning disabilities nurses. This service, unlike that of other paediatric community teams, provides direct care to aid the family in caring for their child either with the family or by acting as a substitute for the family to provide respite from the child's care needs. This can range from overnight care, to day care within the educational environment. Outreach is invariably requested to provide such services because other local resources have not been deemed able to provide direct care for long periods, that is, more than 4 hours.

Open referral system

Telephone/letter to family

Initial assessment

Approach to funding authority for funding

Full assessment

Funding secured and care plan completed with family

Introduction and orientation of Outreach staff to family

Minimum 3 month reviews of service with family and staff

Figure 14.3 Referral process

A 'formalised' referral system was developed (Figure 14.3), although it is effectively an 'open' system so that anyone can refer.

The emphasis is on assessing the child's and family's needs in the community, utilising a care plan format based on Roper's activities of living (1980, cited in Pearson and Vaughan, 1986) to address both the child's and the parent's viewpoints. As a specialised service, the Outreach Service differs from generic paediatric home care services in providing to a wide geographic area – predominantly the southern counties – instead of a specific catchment area.

The Outreach Service model, designed to balance the needs of the children and families and Outreach staff, has been based on four principles; it is:

- focused
- flexible
- friendly
- forward thinking.

Focused

The Outreach Service has focused on children with complex needs and the desire of their families to care for them at home. This has involved matching the necessary skills and expertise from a variety of nursing specialities required to meet the assessed needs of the children and families. The team now consists of an Outreach manager, Outreach liaison nurse, Outreach nurse co-ordinator and a 'bank' of Outreach nursing staff and care assistants. All have the experience of working with children in the community, hospital or school setting. The focus of the service endorses The Children Act 1989 principle that the child's welfare is paramount and that children with disabilities are children with special needs but should be seen as a child first. The child's needs are respected, and where they are able to communicate them, the wishes of the child are taken into account. It has been noted in the past that parents' needs were considered at the expense of the child's (United Nations, 1992). The Outreach Service has developed its own children's charter based on *The Patient's Charter – Services for Children and Young People* (1996) and the United Nations Convention on the Rights of the Child 1992. This is explicit about the standards that can be expected by the children and families who use the service (Figure 14.4).

Outreach staff believe that all children should be accorded full and equal rights.

If you are unable to exercise your rights, Outreach staff will work with you and with your family and others involved in your care, to ensure that your rights are recognised, respected or advocated.

The Outreach staff believes you have a right to:

- be regarded as an individual
- have your best interests considered ao paramount
- be protected from harm
- independence
- privacy
- have your personal dignity respected
- have your emotional, social, cultural and religious needs recognised and respected
- a lifestyle of the highest possible quality
- reach your potential
- have access to any information that affects you
- exercise freedom of choice
- be consulted about your care and contribute to your care plan
- be cared for by appropriately qualified staff in the most appropriate environment
- continuity of care
- the highest possible standard of care
- maintain your interests and friendships
- play and have fun.

Figure 14. 4 Outreach children's charter

CASE STUDY 1

Jane's Outreach Service demonstrates the focused aspect of the service on the child's welfare and needs as being paramount. Jane has severe epilepsy with moderate learning disabilities and associated behaviour problems. The social worker contacted the Outreach Service to request a service when Jane came home from residential school during the holidays. Jane required a carer to be her social model and accompany her to leisure activities, such as swimming, cycling and so on. Jane was able to express what type of carer she wanted to spend her days with, and these wishes were respected and taken into account when matching staff. From the initial assessment, it was considered that a care assistant who had some experience would be suitable. As the service continued, it was felt by the parents and the senior Outreach staff that a qualified nurse with experience with behaviour problems was required. This carer would then be able to deal with any potentially difficult situations, thus instilling Jane's parents with confidence. Jane's seizure pattern became less stable and her behaviour fluctuated, requiring a consistent approach by parents and staff. Jane still had some choice in the staff who cared for her, but the service focused on her needs for skilled staff (Registered Nurse – Learning Disabilities) and her parents' need for reassurance. Jane's parents' experiences of other services had not usually been positive and, over the years, they had tried to cope alone with Jane during school holidays but found this more and more stressful.

The Outreach Service has given Jane and her family the opportunity to enjoy Jane's time at home, which had in the past been unsatisfactory for all the family.

Many of the families Outreach has provided to over the past 2 years have previously had no services focusing on the child with complex needs. This has in turn brought about services that have not provided care when the family needed it or where service providers have not had children's nursing/care experience. The new service has become, therefore, a combination of a nursing agency/community paediatric nursing service purely in the way the service operates, functioning as a licensed nursing agency. However, to the families and children who use the service, it operates as a community paediatric service, providing support and advice in the child's care needs. This is always with the local community team involved, to avoid duplication or confusion.

Flexible

The Outreach Service has developed by responding to the needs of children and families who have been referred to the service, and by the gradual growth in confidence and experience of staff involved. The service has not been prescriptive but has followed a progressive strategy resulting from feedback about the service on evaluation days. These days have enabled parents and staff to discuss both the positive and negative aspects of the service and to seek ways of improving it. The Department of Health's *Welfare of Children and Young People in Hospital* (1991) suggests that there is a need for parents to be fully involved in how services can be developed to meet their needs, not as a paper exercise nor by only paying lip service to consultation. The outcome of the evaluation days and continuous consultation with parents and staff has shown the need for better communication systems, for example mobile phones for key staff, a telephone answering service, a direct line to the service and better information, for example information packs for parents and staff. The need for staff support and training specific to Outreach work has necessitated weekend workshops on areas such as health and safety, and resuscitation in the home. Manual handling training for parents is also planned, as many parents have never had formal training in how to lift correctly or use equipment in the home.

The Outreach Service has proved to be flexible for the families providing all areas of care at the times and in the way the child and family most need it, in many instances preventing hospital admissions. While (1991) suggests that alternatives to hospitalisation have proved attractive on four grounds using paediatric home care services:

1. the reduction of mother and child separation – the avoidance of emotional trauma
2. the decreased anxiety of parents and children
3. the more effective use of resources
4. the reduced incidence of hospital-acquired infection.

CASE STUDY 2

Khalil's Outreach Service demonstrates the above principle of home-based care being an attractive one for the child's welfare and child–parent relationship. Khalil was born with CHARGE association syndrome (Coloboma Heart defects, Atresia of the choanae, Retarded growth, Genital hypoplasia, Ear anomalies and/or deafness) (Contact-a-Family, 1996), spending his first 6 months in a general paediatric unit. His mother desperately wanted to have him at home, but her accommodation was unsuitable and she did not know how she was going to cope by herself with Khalil's care. The local paediatric home care team would have been able to advise and follow up after Khalil's discharge home, but they were not able to provide a day service. The Outreach Service was contacted and asked whether 5 hours of nursing care could be provided in the home once a week. Khalil's mother was rehoused and Khalil came home requiring 24-hour care. At first it proved difficult for both Khalil and his mother to adapt to life at home, although Khalil's mother had excellent support from social services, her general practitioner and the paediatric home care team. The Outreach team worked closely with all involved. In those early months, the Outreach nurse enabled Khalil's mother to sleep, talk about her concerns or go shopping with the confidence that Khalil was being cared for by someone who understood his needs. During the following year, the Outreach Service continued to provide a service when required, for example when Khalil's mother became ill herself and after his discharge from hospital after surgery. The funding authority and Khalil's mother have found the service cost-effective and flexible, meeting Khalil's needs at home in liaison with his local team. Outreach staff were able to provide the expertise to advise on such issues as feeding regimens and stimulation of this child with complex needs.

Khalil's service also highlights the need for appropriate referral and short-term care for children from Asian families, who often do not receive information or home-based respite because of the assumption that the extended Asian family will provide the support. Robina Shah's (1995) investigative study of disabled children in Asian families demonstrated the common false assumptions that these families invariably have the support and help of the extended family. The research shows that, whatever the race or culture, the effect of a child with a disability on the family is no different. It has been the experience of the Outreach Service over the past 2 years to note that there have been referrals from all different parts of the population, especially families from the ethnic minorities. Such family experiences have at times been very negative, this being because of service providers' lack of knowledge of their cultural needs and the assumption that these families do not require outside formal networks of support.

Friendly

The terms 'user-friendly' and 'consumer-friendly' have been overused in recent years and are too often seen only to be paying lip service to the needs of the child, family or staff. In the context of a developing service, the use of 'friendly' as an aspect of the service model for the Outreach Service was seen as essential as it was necessary to be open and receptive to others' views. The aim from the outset was not to be prescriptive but gradually to develop the service around the needs of children and families who used the service, as those needs became apparent. This could only be achieved if open and friendly relationships were developed with families, purchasers and other professionals.

CASE STUDY 3

Jason's Outreach Service will illustrate the 'friendliness' of the 7-nights-a-week service. Jason was born with bronchomalacia and had spent the first 18 months of his life in hospital, with his mother living in with him, becoming an 'expert' in his care. The possibility for Jason to be discharged home depended on the local health authority providing a night service 7 nights a week. Jason's parents felt they could only have him at home if they had the support at night, which would enable them to give their full attention to him during the day. They knew they could not provide his 24-hour care, as he required CPAP (continuous positive airway pressure) ventilation overnight, and monitoring. The health authority approached the Outreach Service, as they did not have the resources to provide such a service themselves. This request came in the first 4 months of the service functioning and was definitely a challenge! The service started off with four nurses providing the service, the 'team' of those able to provide for his needs building up to 12 during the following year. This meant that the margin of safety was sufficient to cope with sickness or other absence. The family and Jason gradually became accustomed to the different staff – not easy when they were trying to adapt to being a family again at the same time. The Outreach team and family built up good communication channels, enabling them to discuss any problems without the fear of being seen to be critical. Unfortunately, many families feel unable to complain about services provided for fear of losing what little support they have. Jason's service has highlighted many areas of development for the service in general, for example staff support groups, staff and parent meetings to discuss future plans of care and the importance of good care plans and documentation of care being provided. The service will gradually decrease as Jason is 'weaned off' his CPAP at night, with an agreed plan between parents, staff and funding authority. This service for Jason and others has proved the importance of the service being seen as approachable and understanding of both family's and staff's needs.

Forward thinking

The service has developed on lines similar to those of other specialised services across the UK, for example The National Assessment Outreach Service for Children with Neuropsychological Disorders. Beale *et al.* (1993) describe how the eventual closure of Hilda Lewis House in Bethlem Royal Hospital, Beckenham, led to the staff's expansion into providing advice and support in the child's own local area. This has been a similar experience for The Children's Trust and staff involved with Outreach. However, unlike the Hilda

Lewis team, the Outreach Service has not come about because of closure but from the perceived and expressed need for flexible care packages. The service has further developmental needs, such as to build-up teams of available staff in the area where a referred child or children live. This will in turn be able to provide the employment of staff who move away from the Trust into other areas of the country, enabling the retention of expertise and skills of staff to meet children's needs across the country. These staff will be seen as key members of satellite teams to be set up in areas expressing an interest in Outreach providing a service to children with complex needs in their area. At the same time, this will enable the service to be more flexible and not require staff to travel long distances.

The service is seeking recognition and accreditation with local authorities and health authorities in order to be seen as credible. It is often expressed by the local authorities, health authorities, education authorities and the independent sector that services are planned collaboratively. The Audit Commission's 1994 report *Seen but not Heard – Co-ordinating Community Health and Social Service for Children* found that children's issues were invariably 'seen but not heard', and it is often the independent sector which, unfettered by the bureaucratic restrictions of the statutory sector, is able to innovate to meet identified needs with a minimum lead time.

CASE STUDY 4

Ann's Outreach Service began when a member of staff went on summer holiday with the family for a week. Ann had contracted meningitis at the age of 18 months, leaving her with learning and physical disabilities. The family had tried a range of services over the years: au pairs, nannies, agency staff and residential respite services. Following the holiday experience, they then requested an after-school service and Saturday service, which was provided by gradually building up a team of staff from her local area over a period of 6 months. In future, a before-school service will be required to enable Ann's mother to take her two other children to two different schools. Ann's service is an example of many others being requested where the Outreach Service is required to provide early morning and after-school services to maintain a child within his or her home and local area. This aspect of the service had not been anticipated, but it can be seen that future demand for this type of provision is likely to increase. To provide for this, the service will require permanent staff who live in the child's local area to provide flexibility, efficiency and continuity.

Conclusion

In conclusion, the Outreach Service has grown rapidly over a 2-year period, and many lessons have been learnt in setting up and providing such a service. It is not a project that should be taken on by others lightheartedly, needing support and commitment from the organisation from which it is provided. The original idea of the service was to release the nursing staff and care staff from the residential units at The Children's Trust. Because of the demand and the geographical distance, the service has needed to be innovative in the area of how to meet this demand, employing ex-Trust staff and staff with the necessary skills in that local area. The service has needed formalised procedures for staff induction, child and family assessments, and the introduction, training and orientation of staff into the child's home to provide a high standard of care. To maintain these standards, there has been a need for the Outreach Service to develop a core team of staff members to manage and deliver the service and to recruit staff to work outside the 9–5 day as most children are within school placements. Due to children in the main not requiring services between 9 am and 5 pm, the Trust has needed to be creative in ways of employing staff working on a zero hour basis, employing staff whose children have grown up and no longer require their presence during the after-school time, and also staff who work in schools during term time and have the school holidays off. The Trust is able to employ them for the children during peak times, which are the school holiday periods.

The service has unlimited potential and has gained a good reputation since its inception. It has the ability to provide a flexible service for families and also flexible working conditions for the staff who provide the service. In addition, it has the ability to provide purchasers with a local service that meets the needs of children with complex requirements working alongside their local community teams. A service like Outreach will continue to grow and develop, based on the service model developed for Outreach. This model will be adapted and changed as the service grows and adapts to the changing care needs of children across the country.

There is clearly a need for evaluation of the Outreach Service. Further research funding will determine, as have other research projects (Burke and Cigno, 1995; Sherman, 1995), the needs of families with a child with a disability/chronic illness and how these services enhance the children's and families' lives.

Sister Frances Dominica suggests that families with children with terminal illness can suffer loneliness and isolation, and require communication, liaison, support and expertise in services provided to them. This is true for all families whose children have complex needs, regardless of whether or not those children are diagnosed as having a life-threatening or life-limiting condition. Outreach staff, as other community staff, can also experience loneliness and feelings of isolation. They too require support in the same way as the people they care for, hence the need for the service to provide a balance between children's, families' and staff's needs.

Key points

The Outreach Service model has aimed to be:

- focused
- flexible
- friendly
- forward thinking
- balanced between the needs of children/parent and staff, all of whom can experience loneliness, isolation and the need for communication, liaison, support and expertise.

References

Audit Commission (1994) *Seen but not Heard: Co-ordinating Community Child Health and Social Services for Children in Need*. (London: HMSO).

Baum, J.D., Dominica, F. and Woodward, R. (1990) *Listen, my Child Has a Lot of Living to Do*. (Oxford: Oxford University Press).

Beale, A. Davies, J., Nixon, J. and Smith, D. (1993) Rising to the challenge. *Nursing Times*, **89**(24): 45–6.

Burke, P. and Cigno, K. (1995) A pilot study on children with learning disabilities and the need for family support. *Health and Social Care in the Community*, **3**: 125–30.

Casey, A., Young, L. and Rote, S. (1997) Integrated nursing services for children. *Paediatric Nursing*, **5**(9): 8.

Contact-a-Family (1996) *The Contact-a-Family Directory of Specific Conditions and Rare Syndromes in Children with their Family Support Networks*, Update 10. (London: Contact-a-Family).

Department of Health (1989) *An Introduction to the Children Act 1989*. (London: HMSO).

Department of Health (1991) *Welfare of Children and Young People in Hospital*. (London: HMSO).

Department of Health (1992) Press Release, *William Waldegrave Announces £5 million Programme to Help Children with Life-threatening Illness.*

Gallagher, A. (1996) Ambulatory care in practice. *Paediatric Nursing,* 8(10): 19–20.

Gould, C. (1996) Multiple partnerships in the community. *Paediatric Nursing,* 8(8): 27–31.

Hubert, J. (1991) *Homebound: Crisis in the Care of Young People with Learning Disabilities.* (London: King's Fund).

Hughes, J. (1997) Reflecting on a community children's nursing service. *Paediatric Nursing,* 9(4): 21–3.

Kelly, P., Taylor, C. and Tatman, M. (1994) Hospital outreach or community nursing? *Paediatric Home Care Child Health,* 2(4): 160–3.

NHS Executive (1996) *A Patients Charter: Services for Children and Young People.* (London: NHSE).

Norah Fry Institute, Russell, O., Macadam, M. and Townsley, R. (1993) *A Study of Likely Future Demand for Specialised Respite Care for Children with Complex Disabilities.* (Bristol: Norah Fry Research Centre).

Pearson, A. and Vaughan, B. (1986) *Nursing Models for Practice.* (London: Heinemann).

Peter, S. and Torr, G. (1996) Paediatric hospital at home the first year. *Paediatric Nursing,* 8(5): 20–3.

Robinson, C. (1995) *Findings from Research on Services to Disabled Children and their Families. Positive Choices: Services for Children with Disabilities.* (London: National Children's Bureau).

Russell, P. (1995) *Positive Choices – Services for Children Living Away from Home.* (London: National Children's Bureau).

Shah, R. (1995) *The Silent Minority: Children with Disabilities in Asian Families,* 2nd edn. (London: National Children's Bureau).

Sherman, B. (1995) Impact on homebased respite care on families and children with chronic illnesses. *Children's Health Care,* 24(1): 33-45.

Tatman, M. and Woodroffe C. (1993) Paediatric home care in the UK. *Archives of Disease in Childhood,* 69: 677–80.

UK Government (1989) *Caring for People: Community Care in the Next Decade and Beyond.* (London: HMSO).

UKHCA (1994) *The United Kingdom Home Care Association Code of Practice.* (Banstead: UKHCA).

United Nations (1992) *The Convention on the Rights of the Child.* (London: HMSO).

While, A. (1991) An evaluation of a paediatric home care scheme. *Journal of Advanced Nursing,* 16: 1413 21.

15

PAEDIATRIC DAY CARE AND ITS CONTRIBUTION TO AMBULATORY CARE NURSING

Lorraine M. Ireland and Helen Rushforth

There is increasing and widespread development of day care services for children. The existence of such services is not new and is founded upon beliefs that relate to the psychological needs of children and their families and also to resource management. Extensive evidence attests to the psychological sequelae of hospitalisation and especially the adverse effects upon those children who are less than 5 years of age. Since the Platt Report (Ministry of Health, 1959), government recommendations have repeatedly emphasised the need, wherever possible, to care for children at home, and if an admission to hospital is required, that this should be for as short a time as possible. Advances in medical technology, anaesthesia and surgical techniques have provided a climate in which it is now possible to obviate the need for overnight stays in hospital for many children.

In considering the terminology, the terms 'day case' and 'day care' seem to be used somewhat interchangeably in the literature. The difference may be one of semantics. However, the trend within the published literature suggests a move from the use of 'day case' towards increasing use of the term 'day care'. This perhaps reflects the earlier emphasis on '*surgical* day *cases*' being replaced by a much broader focus of health *care* encounters. Indeed, Thornes (1991) noted both the continuing confusion over the definition of day cases and the emergence of efforts to widen the category to include *all* ambulatory patients. The current position, as evidenced by this text, suggests that more fluid boundaries are being recognised. However, for the purpose of this chapter, 'day care' is defined as:

the admission of children to hospital for all or part of a day, for the purpose of undergoing surgery, medical therapy, an investigative procedure or observation.

Day care services have historically evolved with considerable diversity in terms of both the environment in which care is delivered and the range of services possible. In 1909, Nicoll (cited by Dearmun, 1994) described surgical procedures that could be undertaken within outpatient clinics. Prior to the evolution of designated beds for day care, such services did exist in other settings; however, the current position endorses a clear commitment to the provision of dedicated day care services. Indeed, there has been a doubling of day case admissions for both medical and surgical care over the period 1989–94. Day case admissions for surgery account for 32.2 per cent of the total number of all paediatric admissions for surgery and for 2.2 per cent of all other paediatric admissions (Moores, 1995).

Thornes (1991), in the report *Just for the Day*, produced by the consortium Caring for Children in the Health Services, highlights the considerable range of day care services that it is possible to provide for children. While each case must clearly be considered individually, and aspects of medical history will on some occasions dictate the need for an inpatient stay (for example for infants born prematurely), the summary given in Table 15.1 indicates a number of common reasons for paediatric day care admission.

Table 15.1 Common reasons for paediatric day care admission

Surgical procedures

General surgery/urology, for example:	Inguinal hernia
	Circumcision
	Orchidopexy
	Cystoscopy
	Manual evacuation
Orthopaedic surgery, for example:	Manipulation
	Change of plaster of Paris
Dental surgery, for example:	Conservation
	Extraction
ENT surgery, for example:	Insertion of grommets
	Examination under anaesthetic
Ophthalmic surgery, for example:	Strabismus (squint) surgery
	Examination under anaesthetic

Plastic surgery, for example: Removal of cysts
                                          Prominent ear correction

Medical procedures

Investigations, for example: Tolerance tests
                                          Jejunal biopsy
                                          CT scans
                                          Renal investigations

Therapy, for example: Administration of immunoglobulin
                                          Blood transfusion

(Based on Thornes, 1991, pp. 13–14).

Opportunities for enhancing care

Day care can offer advantages that are mutually beneficial for families and service providers. The psychological benefits of day care for children and families are widely acknowledged in the literature and can be seen to mitigate the multiple sources of stress for children on entering the hospital system. The reduction in separation of children from their families is perhaps the most widely recognised benefit of day care (Ellerton and Merriman, 1994); indeed, the benefits of maintaining family integrity are conferred not only on the child admitted, but also on the parents and siblings.

The potential for day care to limit the child's exposure to a whole range of frightening experiences and encounters with unfamiliar people cannot be overestimated. Disruption of the child's normal routine is minimised, and a situation is created in which the parent's caring role is not eroded. Once discharged, ongoing recovery takes place in a familiar environment for both parents and child, enabling them to regain mastery and control. It is for all of these reasons that Smith (1991) suggests that day care 'spares children the worst of hospital services'.

Organisationally, day care has numerous advantages for service providers. In maximising the use of health care resources, it has been identified as a way in which costs can be reduced (While and Crawford, 1992; Neill, 1995). These cost savings include those relating to the provision of overnight accommodation, that is, 'hotel services' for children and families. The cost of the admission is also lessened with regard to staffing requirements, notably in unsocial hours payments and in the opportunity to employ part-time staff. Other resource gains are accrued as a result of day care including reduced waiting list time, the liberation of inpatient beds for more complex admissions and a lower incidence of hospital-acquired infection (Brykczynska, 1995; James, 1995). For providers, the potential to offer day care provision is attractive to purchasers, enabling them to compete in the internal health care market.

The clear advantages of day care have been recognised not only by health authorities, but also by the government (While and Crawford, 1992). Health care policies strongly reiterate the case for day care provision. Thornes (1991), in the *Just for the Day* report, identified the 'excellent care' that day services can offer, provided that such services are dedicated exclusively to children's day care. More recently, within the Audit Commission report *Children First* (1993), there is continued endorsement of the development of day care services.

Innovation and excellence in caring – balancing the equation

It can thus be seen that there is a clear mandate to explore and expand the provision of day care services to children, with the aim of enhancing quality of care and reducing the psychological trauma of hospitalisation.

However, there is a danger that financial expediency will drive such innovations faster and further than is in the best interests of the child and family. It is therefore essential to acknowledge the potential difficulties that may exist within day care provision, to ensure that a service is developed that enhances, rather than compromises, the quality of care received.

Significantly, day care places an increased burden of responsibility on the family, who take on the role of 'informal carers' both before and after admission, to a far greater extent than is shouldered by the parents of their inpatient counterparts. Indeed Thornes (1991), in *Just for the Day* explicitly cautions that:

day admissions have to be carefully planned if they are not to cause unnecessary distress to children and their families.

This concern was more recently highlighted within a resolution debated and upheld at RCN Congress (1996). At the heart of the resolution was the concern that expansion of day services has not sufficiently addressed the resulting effects on carers.

Before admission, parents are charged to prepare their child for admission, often necessitating giving explanations of procedures they ill understand themselves. While a number of hospitals run pre-admission programmes, these tend to be surgically focused, to cater for a limited age range and to have variable levels of uptake. Day and inpatient children often attend the same programme, yet the day care families clearly have need of a whole range of specific information; it is perhaps for these families that pre-operative preparation is the most vital (Norris, 1992). In seeking to address such concerns, Dearmun (1994) describes practice in Oxford whereby a senior staff nurse has a joint appointment working between the ward and outpatient settings, providing a key liaison role for the families of children for whom admission is planned.

Pre-operative/procedural fasting is also invariably the remit of day care parents. A range of studies (While and Crawford, 1992; Neill, 1995) demonstrate that day care children are more vulnerable to prolonged starvation, since all children are invariably starved 'as if they were first on the list'. This is further exacerbated by parents tendency to 'overstarve' their children, unaware of the increased risk of nausea, vomiting, hypoglycaemia or failure to pass urine post-procedurally that may result (Neill, 1995). This often causes not only increased distress for the child and family, but also unplanned overnight admission, the very situation that day care sought to avoid. It is also worthy of note that day care families frequently starve themselves alongside their children, further adding to the stress of the day care situation (Norris, 1992).

However, a growing body of evidence is challenging the established fasting times for children. Increasingly shorter fasting times are being advocated (Neill, 1995), which are more realistic for families to comply with, on some occasions even including children receiving a clear drink after admission. Staggered admission times reflecting a predetermined list order are also gradually being adopted. It is important that advice given to parents balances the risk of starving for too long against the risks of not starving for long enough.

Premedication is invariably contraindicated by day surgery, as are longer-acting peri-operative analgesics. There is thus a risk that the benefits of post-operative sedation and pain relief may be lost. While some children require little post-procedural analgesia, a study by Nardone and Schurchiard (1991) suggests that a third of post-operative day cases experience moderate to severe pain. A particular concern is that the expediency of rapid discharge will in some cases

take precedence over the need for premedication or for stronger analgesia because of the prolonging of admission this might entail.

The post-procedural care of children is another area in which
families take a considerable burden of responsibility. Parents and
children alike have a clear need for information to enable them to
manage care following discharge, yet this is an area of day provision that seems frequently to be inadequate (While and Crawford,
1992; Dearmun, 1994; Norinkavitch *et al.*, 1995). Remembering information at times of stress is notoriously difficult, yet day care families are often required to assimilate a range of complex information
in the space of 3 or 4 very stressful hours. They may be required to
observe their child closely with respect to a range of factors, yet
they generally have no nursing expertise. Therefore both written
and verbal information, as well as concrete and unambiguous
'rules' regarding how to interpret any anticipated problems, is paramount. It is essential that the costing and staffing of day care
services recognise that teaching and sharing of information are a
very significant part of the day care nurse's role.

Also fundamental to good day care services is the provision of
ongoing community support for the child and family. Atwell and
Gow (1986) describe setting up one of the earliest paediatric day
surgery units in Southampton in the late 1960s and note the concur-
rent development of a paediatric community nursing service as a
fundamental part of the concept. However, such services remain
relatively scarce, and many children do not receive post-operative
visits (Norris, 1992). In America, home support most usually occurs
in the form of a telephone call, and similar services are being developed in Britain (Freeland and Munro, 1995). Yet studies of day care
repeatedly highlight parents' feelings of vulnerability on discharge
and clear indications that most parents value a home visit (While
and Crawford, 1992; Dearmun, 1994). The current economic climate
within health care provision, however, undermines development of
such services.

Consideration of broader issues relating to day care provision
includes the need to acknowledge the extent to which the informal
carer role that parents adopt is based on informed and voluntary
choice. Thornes (1991) notes the importance of parents only
agreeing to day care following clear explanation and information-
giving, and the opportunity to discuss any concerns. Yet
MacDonald, speaking at the 1996 UK RCN Congress, stated that
parents are in reality often given little choice. Even in situations
where choice is offered, it is difficult to be sure that it can be

achieved in what is often a few very stressful minutes in an outpatients clinic. It is unlikely that many move much beyond coming to terms with the reality of the need for admission, let alone being able objectively to assess the implications of day as opposed to inpatient care. The fact that inpatient waiting lists are often far longer than those for day surgery may be an additional influence on families' compliance (Tasker, 1993). Thus 'negotiation' can become instead 'coercion', a situation that violates the basic principles of family-centred care. It is therefore of vital importance that both medical and nursing staff working in outpatient settings take every step to enable families, as far as possible, to make the decision that is appropriate for them.

Worryingly, day care provision has the potential to become a 'second-class service' (Norris, 1992; Brykczynska, 1995). A particular threat to this becoming a reality is the persistent use of non-dedicated paediatric day services. This may mean children being nursed alongside adults in generic day care facilities. Alternatively, they may be nursed on paediatric inpatient wards and risk being regarded as a 'minor form of inpatient' whose needs may be compromised by those of the 'sicker' children on the ward (Dearmun, 1994). It is for this reason that Thornes (1991) advocates the need for such care to take place in areas designated exclusively for children's day care.

Yet, even within designated day care settings, there is the potential for care to be compromised. Fox (1992) suggests that the introduction of day surgery on a major scale and the accelerated throughput of patients have led to a 'conveyor belt of surgery'. This may lead to an erosion of the provision of nursing care, since such limited time exists for each encounter, and clients may be regarded as having uniform and relatively unproblematic care requirements (Wigens, 1997). This may belie the reality that the families and children who are recipients of day care are a very heterogenous group.

Recognition must also be made that some children admitted for day surgery do not leave the same day. It is inevitable that a small number of children will need to stay overnight, and this should be readily available where it is in their best interest and not regarded as 'failure'. However, the number of children requiring an overnight stay appears to vary enormously, from seven out of ten day cases (While and Crawford, 1992) to seven out of 310 (Tasker, 1993), figures that merit further exploration. There is also an ethical dimension to the overnight stay, in that children's trust may be compromised if they have been assured that they will go home the same day (Brykczynska, 1995). It is a moral requirement that parents and children are aware of the possibility of overnight admission.

Discrimination can also occur in day care provision. A range of factors that influence perceived suitability for day surgery include social class (Thornes, 1991), car and telephone ownership (Tasker, 1993) and being able to speak English (Norinkavitch *et al.*, 1995). Discrimination is likely to be increased if telephone follow-up becomes the norm; while Freeland and Munro (1995) cite the figure of telephone ownership as 87 per cent, this is not evenly distributed between geographical areas or social classes. It is surely essential that all families receive the best possible care and that alternative provision of equal or greater quality is made for those families for whom existing day care arrangements are unsuitable.

Increasing the scope of care

It can thus be seen, that while day care services overall continue to develop, there is far greater emphasis on surgical as opposed to medical provision. However, this may be more apparent than real. The report *Hidden Children* (Thornes, 1988) highlighted that many children receiving medical day care did so as 'ward attenders'. Most of the paediatric units considered within this report did in fact provide day care for medical cases. However, the categorisation of many of these children as 'ward attenders' negated the need for their formal admission, permitting their care to be delivered within already busy and often fully occupied children's wards. Thus these children are less 'visible' than those admitted for surgical interventions. This 'invisibility' of medical day care provision is reinforced by a paucity in the literature, which is almost wholly surgically focused. Thus recognition of the specific and different needs of medical day care families may be lost.

Furthermore, the precedent of associating day care admission with surgery has permitted the evolution of established systems for pre-arranged surgical admissions and greater clarity surrounding the criteria for case selection. In contrast, the criteria for formal admission as a day case for non-surgical intervention is less clear and may be more problematic.

In attempting to address some of these concerns, the Hospitals for Sick Children have set up a 'programmed investigation unit' (PIU) This service takes referrals from all specialities within the medical directorate for children who require a wide range of investigations, with the aim of treating children as day cases wherever possible (Wilks, 1995). This service offers clear benefits for the children and families who would previously have been admitted to busy acute wards and often been considered as of 'low priority'. In establishing this service, nursing staff have been instrumental in developing protocols for care, together with multidisciplinary team members, and have pushed forward the boundaries of their nursing roles.

It is also important to recognise that the characteristics of children undergoing medical day care provision may be dissimilar to those of their surgical counterparts. While some of these medical admissions are healthy and require discrete episodes of care, a large proportion have illness of a chronic or complex nature and will have numerous encounters with health care professionals. For this group, the trajectory of their illness, and therefore their care needs, is very different.

Other innovations in day care move its focus beyond being solely associated with elective admissions. For example, Gallagher (1996) describes an innovation linked to an A&E department, called the 'day assessment unit'. Here, children with a range of problems, such as minor head injuries or some accidental ingestions, can be observed for a few hours and thus usually avoid the need for inpatient admission. The unit will also often admit such children as those with a severe pyrexia or gastroenteritis, thereby allowing a proper assessment to be made over a reasonable time period before deciding whether to admit them or to send them home.

The political climate

It is fundamental to recognise that the provision of day care services has implications for the transfer of costs and medical responsibilities from the hospital to the community and primary care services (Bridger and Rees, 1995).

In the current market-led economy, there is encouragement for diversity and fragmentation between purchasers and providers. Child health care services are supported by a wide range of professionals, each offering a particular body of expertise. Where cross-boundary referrals are made, there can be uncertainty regarding the provision of follow-up post discharge. There is a need for commissioners and providers to collaborate in monitoring the effect of day care provision and allocate resources appropriately.

Atwell and Gow (1985) suggested that day care offered possibilities for 'the integration of hospital and community services'. This possibility needs re-examination in the light of the most recent reform of health care provision in the UK. While some children are nursed in integrated children's Trusts, the majority find their care being split between two or more provider agencies, each of which has its own boundaries. These issues are explored within *Bridging the Gaps* (Thornes, 1993).

Communication with families is potentially compromised when a number of different provider units are involved. Families may be unsure about plans regarding the provision of their health care, and, as Thornes (1993, p. 9) highlighted, 'unsolved issues relating to responsibility, communication and education' may persist. Parent child health records may be one way of addressing this concern, but it must be acknowledged that it will be some time before all children hold such records. In the meantime, there is a more urgent need to develop documentation that bridges the traditional boundaries between hospital and community, and also between professionals and carers. Without such developments, there is a very real risk that the standards in the *Children's Charter* (Department of Health, 1996) regarding discharge planning could become more rhetoric than reality.

This fragmentation also has a more general impact on care management and delivery. Financial implications of care being delivered by two different Trusts may mean that both try to incur minimum expenditure within their own budget and are reluctant to take on any responsibilities beyond their immediate sphere of practice. This belies a reality that children undergoing day care inevitably cross boundaries; there is the potential for this fragmentation to undermine the development of a 'seamless' service. Furthermore, such financial constraints stifle the development of new services; currently, only 50 per cent of districts have a dedicated paediatric community nursing service (Burr, 1996). In addition to conflict between hospital and community Trusts, Bridger and Rees (1995) point out that fundholding general practitioners are also increasingly picking up the cost of day care; they cite figures by Scott (1992) which suggest that a third of all individuals who receive day care consult their general practitioner as a direct result within the following 7 days. It would be interesting to correlate these findings with the provision of post-procedural community nursing follow-up.

One way of addressing some of the challenges that day care presents is by taking a more explicit approach to multidisciplinary care management and communication. Integrated care pathways have been identified as one way of achieving these goals. They facilitate the synchronisation of nursing, medical and paramedical activities in order to ensure that clients receive optimal care from experts in each discipline (Johnson, 1994). Such pathways can be very sophisticated, incorporating protocols, standards and audit measures. One step towards this is the development of a 'unitary patient record', where all care is planned and recorded in a common document. An example of this is the documentation used by the day care service at the Royal Alexandra Hospital for Sick Children in Brighton. The record forms the basis of a nurse-led clerking service, which maximises continuity of care and minimises the number of health care practitioners with whom families come into contact.

The political agenda to decentralise services and increase local health care initiatives is reflected in Thornes (1991, 1993). While the value to families of having local day care provision is clear, a balance needs to be achieved between geographical location and the provision of expertise. Traditionally, much paediatric surgery has been located in regional centres, where surgical and anaesthetic expertise is arguably at its greatest. However, political and financial pressures mean that a growing number of day surgery cases in particular are being undertaken in 'satellite centres', often by general surgeons and anaesthetists who inevitably have less paediatric expertise. The overt attraction of a local service may thus belie the reality that such a service may be of a lower standard than that which a regional centre can provide. It is therefore important that general practitioners and other purchasers have knowledge of the expertise and facilities available. There is also a growing trend among a number of fundholding general practitioners to push forward the scope of the surgical procedure that they perform within their own practice settings; arguably, financial expediency influences such decisions. Although this has as yet mostly affected adult clients, it is not difficult to conceive of a situation in which minor paediatric services might follow a similar pattern.

Processes of decentralisation have also led to a situation whereby a growth in the number of services providers has led to a potential underutilisation of day care facilities. This challenges providers to diversify in order to maximise bed occupancy. It is therefore opportune to consider the incorporation of medical day care services, investigation units and assessment units, as earlier discussed, into existing day care settings.

There is a need within care provision 'for all concerned to accept an agreed standard of care, and to ensure that the child is in the right place to receive it' (Thornes, 1993, p. 22). An example of good practice in this respect is demonstrated by the North West Region Benchmarking Group (Ellis, 1996). Practitioners who have involvement in a diverse range of day care services throughout the northwest of England regularly meet together to discuss factors that allow the provision of best practice, identifying these from practice examples, practice-based research and professional consensus. This leads to the development of a 'benchmark' statement that defines best practice, central to which is effective multidisciplinary working. Examples of this approach include the organisation of dedicated paediatric theatre lists and the use of individualised multidisciplinary care pathways. Practitioners can make a comparison of practice with others, sharing problems or successes and supporting each other in achieving optimum standards of care. For example, they may have had similar problems in establishing well-attended and effective pre-admission clinics, or in compiling multilingual information leaflets. They can share their solutions and, hopefully, prevent wastage of resources and 'reinventing the wheel'.

Conclusion

It can thus be seen that the development of paediatric day care provision is one which offers many opportunities to enhance the care that the child and family receive. While importantly, those aspects of day care where quality of care may be compromised are acknowledged, there is also much evidence of ongoing research and practice innovation that is seeking to address these concerns and work towards care delivery of the highest standard.

In summary, therefore, the following is offered, as 'guidelines for good practice in paediatric day care provision'.

GUIDELINES FOR GOOD PRACTICE IN PAEDIATRIC DAY CARE PROVISION

- A commitment by all providers of paediatric day care provision to offer a dedicated service that is set up exclusively for this client group.

- The further development of day care services for minor medical procedures, treatments and investigations currently carried out on a inpatient basis.

- Enhanced data collection regarding those children currently described as 'ward attenders' in order that they can be made more explicit within calculations of costing and care provision.

- An increasing awareness among all health care practitioners of the need fully to assess the appropriateness of day care provision for each child and family, and a commitment to open negotiation and collaborative decision-making that is in their best interest.

- That tertiary centres explore possibilities of working together with local services to provide 'shared care', whereby not only outpatient visits but also pre-procedural preparation and even pre-clerking might take place locally, thereby minimising the disruption to the family of travelling repeatedly to the tertiary centre.

- A commitment to giving families information to allow them to prepare adequately for their child's day care. This includes:
  - sufficient information regarding the nature of the procedure and the day of admission
  - the opportunity to receive formal pre-admission preparation
  - clear guidance for the family regarding the purposes and duration of fasting.

- Current research findings regarding the time needed for pre-procedural fasting will be reinforced by larger-scale inquiry and used to inform practice in order to minimise the distress caused to children and their families by prolonged starvation.

- An audit of pain experienced by children undergoing day procedures, and the development of pain management that recognises the needs of this specific client group.

- The provision of verbal and written information for all families regarding day care procedures, which enables them to carry out ongoing care effectively. This should include clear guidelines regarding the interpretation of post-procedural symptoms that the child may exhibit following discharge, and at what point to seek professional help and from whom.

- The provision of predetermined community support that reflects the families' needs and wishes. At a broader political level, a enhanced commitment to the need for all children to have access to a paediatric trained community nurse.

- Greater collaboration between service providers in hospital and community settings, with the aim of providing a 'seamless' service. Also collaboration between service providers in different acute Trusts to facilitate shared learning, professional consensus and achievement of the highest possible standards of care.

References

Atwell, J.D. and Gow, M.A. (1985) Paediatric trained district nurses in the community: expensive luxury or economic necessity? *British Medical Journal*, **291**: 227–9.

Audit Commission (1993) *Children First: A Study of Hospital Services.* (London: HMSO).

Bridger, P. and Rees, M. (1995) What a difference a day makes. *Health Service Journal*, **105**: 22–3.

Brykczynska, G. (1995) Ethics of day surgery for children. *Surgical Nurse,* 8(1): 11–13.

Burr, S. (1996) Editorial: Children's services still inadequate – 37 years on. *Paediatric Nursing,* 8(3): 3.

Dearmun, A. (1994) Defining differences: children's day surgery. *Surgical Nurse,* 7(6): 7–11.

Department of Health (1996) *The Patient's Charter: Services for Children and Young People.* (London: HMSO).

Ellerton, M. and Merriman, C. (1994) Preparing children and families psychologically for day surgery: an evaluation. *Journal of Advanced Nursing,* 19: 1057–62.

Ellis, J. (1996) Benchmarking in paediatrics. Paper presented at the Association of British Paediatric Nurses Annual Conference, April.

Fox, N. (1992) *The Social Meaning of Surgery.* (Milton Keynes: Open University Press).

Freeland, A.M. and Munro, K.M. (1995) All part of the service. *Child Health,* 3(4): 154–8.

Gallagher, A. (1996) Ambulatory care in practice. *Paediatric Nursing,* 8(10): 19–20.

James, J. (1995) Day care admissions. *Paediatric Nursing,* 7(1): 25–37.

Johnson, S. (1994) Patient focused care without the upheaval. *Nursing Standard,* 8(29): 20–2.

Ministry of Health (1959) *Welfare of Children in Hospital* (Platt Report). (London: HMSO).

Moores, Y. (1995) The challenge ahead. *Child Health,* 3(4): 131–5.

Nardone, P. and Schurchiard, B. (1991) Parental pain perception of the same day pediatric patient. *Journal of Nursing Quality Assurance,* 5(3): 59–64.

Neill, S. (1995) Fasting for day surgery: the parental role. *Paediatric Nursing,* 7(2): 20–3.

Norinkavich, K., Howie, G. and Cariofiles, P. (1995) Quality improvement study of day surgery for tonsillectomy and adenoidectomy patients. *Pediatric Nursing (US),* 21(4): 341–4.

Norris, E. (1992) Care of the paediatric day-surgery patient. *British Journal of Nursing,* 1(11): 547–51.

RCN (1996) UK Annual Congress, *Resolution 10,* 23 April, Bournemouth.

Smith, J. (1991) Editorial: Children could benefit from an expansion in day care services in British hospitals. *Journal of Advanced Nursing,* 16: 767–8.

Tasker, M. (1993) Day case adenoidectomy for children. *Paediatric Nursing,* 5(2): 18–19.

Thornes, R. (1988) *Hidden Children.* (London: National Association for the Welfare of Children in Hospital).

Thornes, R. (1991) *Just for the Day.* (London: National Association for the Welfare of Children in Hospital).

Thornes, R. (1993) *Bridging the Gaps.* (London: Action for Sick Children).

While, A. and Crawford, J. (1992) Paediatric day surgery. *Nursing Times,* 88(39): 43–5.

Wigens, L. (1997) The conflict between 'new nursing' and 'scientific management' as perceived by surgical nurses. *Journal of Advanced Nursing,* 25: 1116–22.

Wilks, Z. (1995) A better way of testing. *Charter News,* 9: 6–7.

16

AMBULATORY CARE FOR CHILDREN WITH NEWLY DIAGNOSED DIABETES

Lesley Lowes and Ruth Davis

Childhood diabetes

Type 1 or insulin-dependent diabetes mellitus (IDDM) is one of the most common chronic childhood disorders, the incidence for children aged under 15 years in the British Isles almost doubling from 7.7/100 000 per year in 1973–74 to 13.5/100 000 per year in 1988 (Metcalfe and Baum, 1991). The lack of insulin production in IDDM results in high blood glucose levels (hyperglycaemia), leading to increased micturition by day and night, sometimes with uncharacteristic bedwetting, increased thirst, fatigue and weight loss. If undetected, severe fluid, electrolyte and acid base disturbances lead to vomiting, dehydration, coma and death. The presentation at diagnosis can vary considerably, from the acutely ill, ketoacidotic child with severe dehydration to the relatively asymptomatic child where the disease has been recognised in the early stages of its development.

The medical interventions necessary to stabilise newly diagnosed diabetes depend upon the clinical condition of the child at presentation. An initial period of hospitalisation is necessary if intravenous therapy is required to correct dehydration, electrolyte imbalance and ketoacidosis, with progression to oral fluids and subcutaneous insulin administration as the child's clinical condition improves. If the child is asymptomatic, or mildly to moderately symptomatic and clinically well, subcutaneous insulin and oral diet and fluids may be commenced from diagnosis. Treatment regimens vary according to local protocols and preferences, but children are commonly started on an initial regimen of twice-daily injections of insulin in conjunction with a healthy diet that restricts the intake of sugary foods. Blood glucose monitoring may initially be performed up to four times a day before meals, with more frequent monitoring as necessary, such as during periods of acute illness.

Impact of diagnosis

The literature widely supports the view that the diagnosis of IDDM in childhood is disruptive to family life (Baum, 1990; Pinkney *et al.*, 1994), exacting a physical and emotional toll on both children and families. Diabetes management requires a detailed and lifelong commitment to a complex treatment regimen, balancing insulin dosage with the child's dietary requirements and daily level of activity. In the short term, the family have to cope with the initial acute stage of this chronic disease, while grieving for the loss of their healthy child. Parental decisions about everyday issues and usual childhood activities, such as school, swimming with friends, going to birthday parties and particularly diet, take on a different perspective for the family whose child has diabetes. Life events and stressors will alter glycaemic control, demanding various coping strategies by children and families as they struggle to maintain good control of the diabetes in order to sustain good health, promote growth and development, and prevent or minimise the risk of the complications of diabetes in later life.

Starting treatment: hospital versus home

Children's vulnerability to the emotional impact of illness and hospitalisation is well recognised, resulting in a firm belief that the minimisation or avoidance of hospitalisation is in children's best interests (Department of Health, 1991; Royal College of Nursing, 1994). The Department of Health (1991) recommends that children should only be admitted to hospital if the appropriate care cannot be provided in the community. Viointainer and Wolfer (1975) identi fied some of the features of hospital that can worry a child, including physical harm/bodily injury, separation from parents, the strange and unknown, the possibility of surprise, uncertainty about limits and expected 'acceptable' behaviour, and the relative loss of control, autonomy and competence. Studies undertaken to examine the psychological effect of hospitalisation on children show a range of factors which may influence any particular child's short- or long-term reaction. These include the reason for the admission, any previous experience of illness or hospital, the child's age and psychological make-up, stressful events prior to hospitalisation, whether parent–child separation occurs, the parental reaction during and after the period of hospitalisation and the extent of preparation for admission (McClowry and McLeod, 1990; Muller *et al.*, 1994). However, there is a general consensus of opinion that younger children show greater adverse reactions to hospitalisation, such as aloofness towards their parents, clinging or demanding behaviour, withdrawal, hyperactivity, food finickiness, skill regression, night waking and fear of separation from their parents. Older children appear to cope better with the experiences of hospital (Visintainer and Wolfer, 1975; McClowry and McLoed, 1990), but while they may be more resilient to the stresses of hospitalisation, any apparent lack of reaction may be due to an ability to disguise their feelings (McClowry and McLeod, 1990).

The good control of childhood diabetes is ultimately dependent on the competence and management ability of the child/family, and the development of the necessary management skills may be facilitated through active, practical involvement of the child/family from diagnosis (Swift *et al.*, 1993). If the child is clinically well, this may be accomplished more effectively in the home environment, where nursing input is predominantly educative and supportive, than in a ward environment, where families may feel less in control and more likely to become dependent on the interventions of others. The comparative lack of privacy in hospital may also inhibit families from sharing the grief that is believed to accompany the diagnosis of diabetes and other chronic illnesses. The expression of emotional pain may facilitate parental adjustment, if it represents a way of 'working through' towards acceptance of the diagnosis, and it is possible that parents and their children would feel more able to share their feelings, experiencing any initial trauma together, in the privacy of their own home.

In hospital, the diabetes is stabilised according to the child's activity level and dietary intake on the ward. These may differ greatly from the child's normal activity and diet at home, and may result in a loss of glycaemic control and feelings of failure among the family if problems arise after discharge. With home management, stabilisation occurs in the child's normal environment, the necessary adjustments of insulin being based on the child's usual lifestyle, near normal activities and dietary intake. It seems reasonable that variability of control is better understood when explained practically in the context of familiar, everyday occurrences, enabling the family to anticipate preventative or corrective measures in the future.

At a time when family support is imperative, hospitalisation often results in the separation of partners and siblings. In a two-parent family, the responsibility for the child's health typically falls on the mother (Moyer, 1989), and the onus is often on her to develop an understanding of the various aspects of diabetes management and convey these to other family members. In this situation, feelings of isolation by both partners may result, with fathers and siblings feeling left out and unable to participate fully if the education is aimed at the mother. Educational involvement and the active participation of both parents from the time of diagnosis, whether in hospital or at home, should therefore be encouraged, a view supported by Anderson et al. (1983), whose study found that participation in diabetes management skills by both parents in two-parent families resulted in the child having significantly better overall control.

Families with complex family commitments may find that initial hospitalisation provides a less demanding environment to facilitate the learning process, giving parents time to come to terms with the diagnosis, develop an understanding of IDDM and learn the necessary practical skills, while the initial diabetes management is undertaken by hospital staff. However, hospitalisation may result in increased stress if essential domestic arrangements, such as the care of siblings, are difficult to organise, particularly in the case of single-parent families or those without extended family support. In this context, the benefits of home management for three individual families are described by McEvilly (1991), in which the complications of new born or handicapped siblings and an absent father would have made hospitalisation difficult.

Additional factors in favour of ambulatory care were found in the study by Swift et al. (1993). They found lower readmission rates in a non-hospitalised group of children, and although they could not conclusively prove cause and effect, they concluded that home management was the most probable reason.

One of the outcomes of home management and minimal hospitalisation is the reduction in bed occupancy (Swift et al., 1993). This has implications for improved cost-effectiveness, as long as the services that are put in its place are not more expensive. In the USA, Lipman (1987) calculated that a mean 2-day reduction in length of stay represented a saving of $538 a day for room and board, but there was no reference to the cost of any contributing interventions, such as additional community or specialist nursing services. When evaluating the effects of home management, the needs of the child and family should be paramount, but financial implications have to be considered in the resource-constrained climate of contemporary health care. The costs of care in chronic disease are complex and multifaceted. Few studies have fully addressed the costs of this treatment option, and more are needed to look at the clinical and cost-effectiveness of the services being provided.

An increasing awareness of the psychological (Department of Health, 1991) and economic benefits of home care and minimal hospitalisation is reflected in the recent downward trend in the length of children's hospitalisation in England and Wales (Royal College of Nursing, 1994). The RCN (1994) recommend that, to enable children to be cared for in their own homes, support should be provided by the creation of paediatric community services or through paediatric clinical nurse specialists who work in the hospital and the community, specialising in a particular condition.

Initial management in the British Isles

Historically, children with newly diagnosed diabetes, regardless of their clinical condition, have been routinely admitted for the initial management of their diabetes, often hospitalised for longer than a week (Lessing et al., 1992). Prior to the availability of the necessary equipment for home blood glucose monitoring, newly diagnosed children required hospitalisation for laboratory testing of blood glucose levels. An initial period of hospitalisation continues to be widespread practice (British Paediatric Association Working Party Report, 1990), to the extent that 96 per cent of children under 15 years of age living in the British Isles who were diagnosed in 1988 were admitted to hospital at the time of diagnosis (Lessing et al., 1992). Factors that contribute to the low percentage of children who are managed at home from diagnosis include family doctors who delay or do not contact the diabetes team, a lack of local resources for home care, a belief by diabetes teams that hospitalisation is necessary for effective early management and perhaps an unquestioning adherence to traditional management methods. A survey of British paediatricians (British Paediatric Association Working Party Report, 1990) found that, while 87 per cent admitted more than 80 per cent of all newly diagnosed children, 47 per cent would change this policy if better services were available in the community. While there are no large-scale studies to confirm the trend, it is likely that the number of children managed as outpatients at diagnosis is rising. This may be due to the increasing emphasis on paediatric community care, the potentially adverse effects of hospitalisation for children (Department of Health, 1991; Royal College of Nursing, 1994) and/or the belief that it is more cost-effective to maintain a chronically ill child at home (Royal College of Nursing, 1994).

Outpatient management of children with newly diagnosed diabetes is not a recent innovation. Swift et al. (1993) report on Walker's work in Leicestershire in the early 1950s. Out of 136 children diagnosed between 1950 and 1966, only 35 referred directly to the diabetic clinic were admitted to hospital. More recently, over a 10-year period from 1979 to 1988, only 98 (42 per cent) out of a total of 236 newly diagnosed children in Leicestershire were admitted at diagnosis, with only 60 per cent of those admitted requiring intravenous therapy. The mean duration of hospitalisation decreased from 7 to 3 days over the same period. Since 1988, over 80 per cent of newly diagnosed children in Leicestershire have been managed as outpatients, community care being undertaken by specialist diabetes health visitors, assisted by community nurses. Swift et al. (1993) directly attribute the success of total home management to the availability and commitment of a specialist paediatric diabetes team.

However, other study findings do not show the high percentage of outpatient management demonstrated in Leicestershire, some areas routinely admitting all newly diagnosed children. Wearmouth (1994), in a review of 101 children diagnosed between 1982 and 1990 at Poole General Hospital, found that all newly diagnosed children were admitted for initial treatment and education, although there was a consistent downward trend in the length of inpatient stay (from a mean of 14.3 days to one of 8.0). Wearmouth concluded that the reduction in length of stay reflected changing attitudes to community-based management, although he believes that there may also be a possible association with families having a history or prior knowledge of IDDM.

A study undertaken by Pinkney et al. (1994) surveyed 230 patients under 21 years of age from the Oxford Regional Health Authority who had diabetes diagnosed in 1985/86, and compared their clinical presentation and management with a second cohort of 97 similar patients diagnosed in 1990. The results found that the rates of admission at diagnosis (79 per cent admitted), did not differ between the two cohorts of patients, those admitted being significantly younger than those not admitted, although the mean age at diagnosis was significantly lower in the 1990 cohort (9.4 years compared with 12.4 years in 1985/86). Ketoacidosis of any degree was most common in children below five years of age, becoming less common with increasing age. Almost half of those managed as outpatients (48 per cent) occurred in two of the eight districts surveyed, although no reason was given for local variance in management. Pinkney *et al.* stated that the majority of paediatricians in the Oxford Region admitted at diagnosis, unless the family had previous knowledge of IDDM, but the mean duration of length of stay for children was not mentioned. The study findings suggested that admission at diagnosis did not affect subsequent outcome measures, such as readmission or episodes of severe hypoglycaemia, even when the groups were matched for severity of disease at presentation.

There is some evidence in the literature of an increasing trend towards reducing the length of hospitalisation for newly diagnosed children. In Cardiff, the introduction of home management, facilitated by input from a newly appointed paediatric diabetes specialist nurse, has achieved a significant reduction in length of stay for children with newly diagnosed diabetes (Cowan *et al.*, 1997; Lowes, 1997; Lowes and Davis, 1997). Similarly, the establishment of a Diabetic Home Care Unit at Birmingham Children's Hospital in 1981 reduced inpatient stay from an average of 10 days in 1980 to 2 days in 1990, some children subsequently receiving total home management (McEvilly, 1991).

The above studies highlight significant differences in practice in initial management methods and the length of a child's hospitalisation at diagnosis over a similar period of time. Findings from these studies seem to suggest that hospitalisation is minimised or avoided when children with newly diagnosed diabetes are looked after by a specialist paediatric diabetes team with the appropriate community resources. Diabetes specialist nurses appear to play a major part in reducing hospitalisation and facilitating home management, by continuing the care and management of newly diagnosed children and their families in the home environment (McEvilly, 1991; Lowes and Davis 1997), providing frequent telephone contacts and home/outpatient visits with support from other members of the diabetes team.

Diabetes world wide

Hospitalisation for children with newly diagnosed diabetes is common world wide, but the issue of reducing or eliminating hospital stays is being widely debated. It is difficult to generalise about care in the USA, but several centres have described their experiences of eliminating unnecessary hospitalisation and some now have many years experience (Schneider, 1983; Hamman *et al.*, 1985).

In Japan, the average length of hospitalisation is 3 weeks (Koizumi, 1992). In Finland it is 4 weeks, although Simell *et al.* (1993) demonstrated that the length of stay could be reduced from a mean of 23 days to 9 days without an effect on metabolic or psychosocial outcome and with a cost saving of 36 per cent. In Sweden, Forsander (1995) estimated the average length of hospitalisation as being 3 weeks. In a prospective randomised study involving early discharge to a training apartment, he showed improvements in information and attention received and also in the emotional response to treatment.

The role of the paediatric diabetes specialist nurse

Over the past two decades, the nursing care of children with diabetes has largely come under the remit of diabetes specialist nurses who have combined both adult and paediatric care, sometimes finding difficulty in justifying the disproportionate amount of time spent with the children, who form a very small part of their caseload (McEvilly, 1995). However, the role of the diabetes specialist nurse caring for children differs from that of the adult diabetes specialist nurse, not because of the diabetes but because of the needs of the client population. The paediatric diabetes specialist nurse has a responsibility not only to care for and educate the child with diabetes, but also to educate and support parents, the extended family, teachers and others on whom the child will depend. During term time, nursery and school-age children spend a large part of the day away from their parents. To support the teachers, reassure the parents and minimise the risk to the children, the paediatric diabetes specialist nurse provides school visits with education for the professionals and other carers who share responsibility for the children.

In recognition of the need to develop a body of knowledge about the diabetes specialist nurse role, function and approach to care, Moyer (1993) undertook a 12-month community-based study exploring specialist nursing care for children with diabetes. Findings from this study highlighted the multifaceted role of diabetes specialist nurses, the flexibility of which enabled them to cross the boundary between hospital and community, providing integrated and consistent care. Effective, often long-term, nurse–child–family relationships had been established, which facilitated the provision of support and education by diabetes specialist nurses, in times of illness and health, to families of newly diagnosed children and those with established diabetes. Strategies aimed at achieving the three main goals of optimal metabolic control, responsible self-care and a normal life were situation specific and tailored to children's individual needs, depending on the child's age, the diabetic condition and life events. While developing the expertise of children towards these goals, the diabetes specialist nurses worked simultaneously with parents and others, addressing some of the many health and/or developmental problems in relation to diabetes management, to create an environment that supported attainment of these goals.

Following the Allitt Inquiry (Department of Health, 1994) guidelines for paediatric nursing care were reviewed, increased emphasis being placed on the recommendation that nurses caring for children should be Child Branch (Project 2000) or Registered Sick Children's Nurses (Royal College of Nursing, 1994). This would ensure that children were looked after by appropriately trained health professionals who had the knowledge and skills to meet the specific needs of children and their families. Effective education is essential to successful diabetes management and the maintenance of good health in diabetes. When the recipients are children and their families, the diabetes specialist nurse needs to have a knowledge of child development, an understanding of children's special needs and an ability to understand the problems of diabetes management from the perspectives of both the child and the parents. As children develop and cognitive abilities increase, their educative requirements change, so that diabetes education is an ongoing process throughout childhood and adolescence.

The role of the diabetes specialist nurse has been outlined in an RCN working party report (Royal College of Nursing Paediatric Diabetes Special Interest Group, 1993). In practice, the variability and extent of the paediatric diabetes specialist nurse role may be influenced by local organisation of services, caseload numbers, the size of the nursing team and the method of diabetes management employed at diagnosis, with individually defined job specifications for any particular post. The key worker with children with diabetes and their families, particularly in the community setting, is often identified as the paediatric diabetes specialist nurse who contributes significantly, as a member of a specialist diabetes team, to the facilitation of home management for newly diagnosed children (Swift *et al.*, 1993; McEvilly, 1995). As the paediatric diabetes specialist nurse provides the bulk of care, advice and support in the early days, flexibility of working hours may be necessary to meet the immediate needs of the newly diagnosed child and family. Where home management is a practised approach to initial care, there is a belief that parents require 24-hour accessibility to the diabetes team (Lowes and Davis, 1997), and the paediatric diabetes specialist nurse may often be involved in the provision of this service. Several approaches to providing 24-hour access to the diabetes team have been described. McEvilly (1991) describes a team of nurses, whereas Swift *et al.* (1993) and Lowes and Davis (1997) report the use of members of the diabetes team with hospital back-up.

Starting treatment: clinical practice

CASE STUDY 1
UNIVERSITY HOSPITAL OF WALES
HEALTHCARE NHS TRUST, CARDIFF

Approaches to the practical organisation of home management will vary according to local protocols and resources, and to give a more detailed illustration, the care of newly diagnosed children by the paediatric diabetes team at the University Hospital of Wales, Cardiff, will be discussed. This multidisciplinary team cares for 160 children with diabetes, with approximately 21 newly diagnosed children each year. In paediatric diabetes care, an integrated team approach in which individual roles are recognised and respected is essential. This promotes effective communication within the team, facilitating consistent advice to children and their families and reducing feelings of isolation by individual team members. In Cardiff, team meetings and clinical audit are held twice a year to discuss, evaluate and improve the effectiveness of service provision. Team members include a consultant paediatric endocrinologist, a lecturer in child health, a paediatric dietitian, a paediatric senior registrar, a clinical assistant, a growth nurse specialist, a paediatric diabetes specialist nurse, two diabetes specialist nurses (with adult and paediatric caseloads), a clinical child psychologist and a social worker. The paediatric diabetes specialist nurse cares specifically for children, undertaking primary nursing responsibility for the home management of newly diagnosed children as part of her role. An integrated approach to care in hospital and community settings allows the paediatric diabetes specialist nurse to provide a seamless package from diagnosis.

With the appointment of the paediatric diabetes specialist nurse in April 1995, a protocol for the home management of children with newly diagnosed diabetes was devised and implemented in August 1995. All children presenting with newly diagnosed diabetes are assessed on the paediatric unit, and there are clearly defined criteria for identifying those children who can safely be managed at home. Home management from diagnosis is instigated if the child is assessed by the medical staff to be clinically well (without significant acidosis) and the appropriate members of the paediatric diabetes team, including the paediatric diabetes specialist nurse, are available. Other relevant factors include the preference of individual families, the child's age, other family commitments, access to a telephone and psychosocial issues, such as the family's initial reaction to the diagnosis.

If hospitalisation is necessary, the paediatric diabetes specialist nurse, where possible, meets the child and family on the day of diagnosis. Initial support and diabetes education are provided by the nursing staff on the ward in conjunction with the paediatric diabetes specialist nurse. Home management and the minimal hospitalisation of children with diabetes has the potential to deskill ward-based nurses. To avoid this, bi-monthly diabetes seminars and informal teaching sessions are organised by the paediatric diabetes specialist nurse, to enable ward nurses to remain up to date in the area of diabetes management. Dietary advice from the paediatric dietitian begins in hospital and, following discharge, continues in the paediatric diabetes clinic. The child is discharged home as soon as possible, with support and diabetes education continued by the diabetes specialist nurses, who commence home visits on the day of discharge, their frequency and number depending on individual family needs.

When home management is considered to be appropriate, the paediatric diabetes specialist nurse introduces herself to the child and family in the paediatric emergency assessment unit before their discharge home. Insulin therapy is prescribed by the medical staff and is instigated at home, usually within hours of the diagnosis, by the paediatric diabetes specialist nurse, who, for the first few days, will liaise with her medical colleagues about any adjustment of insulin dosage. As nursing roles change with the development of services such as home management, issues of interprofessional accountability will arise. It has been recognised that there is an urgent need for clarification of the legal situation concerning prescribing by nurses (Royal College of Paediatrics and Child Health and the Joint British Advisory Committee on Children's Nursing, 1996), who may be particularly vulnerable if decisions about the adjustment of medication are an integral part of their role. It is vital that, within multidisciplinary diabetes teams, there are effective channels of communication with easy accessibility to appropriate team members, and that diabetes specialist nurses are adequately supported by their medical colleagues. This is an important consideration, as the relative autonomy of this specialist nurse role can result in feelings of isolation and ultimate responsibility for the welfare of the newly diagnosed child. In Cardiff, before home management was implemented, guidelines for insulin adjustment were clarified by the consultant paediatrician, and the diabetes specialist nurses are able to contact one of their medical colleagues at any time for decisions about the adjustment of insulin or advice about any aspect of the diabetes management.

Home visits are carried out up to four times a day initially to provide emotional support and education about diabetes and to teach and supervise the practical skills of blood glucose monitoring and insulin administration. The frequency of home visits is dependent on the individual needs of any particular family, continuity and consistency of care being provided via a shared care approach by the diabetes specialist nurses. At the time of diagnosis, children and their families are given a simple explanation about the altered physiology in diabetes in order to help them understand the need for insulin replacement. The association between insulin administration and hypoglycaemia is also explained. Simple dietary guidelines are outlined: the importance of regular meals, the avoidance of sugary food and drinks and the inclusion of carbohydrate in every meal and snack, with a list of appropriate basic foods. A booklet about diabetes, designed for children and their families (Paediatric Diabetes Teams, Newcastle and Gateshead, 1993), is issued on the day of diagnosis, to allow families to begin the learning process in their own time. The rate of progress through the education programme depends on the level of understanding for each individual family, and while it is important to ensure that families have received essential information, they should not be overloaded. At this stage, children and their families may be unable to retain information because of the shock of diagnosis, feelings of grief and natural anxiety, so all information given needs to be repeated and reinforced at a later date. Other topics covered in the education programme include information about insulin, the avoidance, recognition and treatment of hypoglycaemia and hyperglycaemia, the management of illness, the importance and effect of exercise, and other diabetes-related issues, such as personal identification, benefits and the services available.

The hospital-based paediatric dietitian undertakes the dietary component of the education programme on an outpatient basis but is also available for immediate advice during working hours. Families are given written dietary advice emphasising healthy eating for the family as a whole, with a realistic, individual approach to suggested eating plans incorporating foods usually eaten by the family. Feeding the newly diagnosed child appears to be one of the major concerns for families in the early days, so basic guidelines are provided using the exchange system (1 exchange = 10 g carbohydrate). The dietitian works closely with other members of the paediatric diabetes team, giving consistent advice about the treatment of hypoglycaemia, the management of exercise, carbohydrate intake during illness, eating out, food labelling and food preparation.

When the newly diagnosed child and/or parents demonstrate an under-standing of diabetes management and are able to carry out the neces-sary practical skills, home visits are reduced in agreement with the wishes of individual families. Education is continued and support main-tained through less frequent home visits, telephone contact and clinic visits, with the child and family attending the next available paediatric diabetes clinic following diagnosis. The paediatric diabetes specialist nurse, consultant paediatrician and lecturer in child health provide ongoing support from 8 am until midnight for all children and their fami-lies under the care of the paediatric diabetes service, using a portable telephone and long-range paging system. Overnight, families are able to telephone the paediatric ward staff for help and advice; the ward staff will, if necessary, contact the consultant paediatrician at home.

As soon as possible after diagnosis, the diabetes specialist nurses contact other professionals who are involved in the care of the newly diagnosed child. These may include childminders and nursery or school teachers, to whom education about the relevant aspects of diabetes management is offered. This gives parents the confidence to allow their children safely and speedily to resume their usual daily activities, promoting 'normality' for the family as a whole. Many school-aged, newly diagnosed children return to full-time education within a few days of diagnosis.

Starting treatment: research-based evidence for minimising hospitalisation

As previously outlined, one of the main aims of the paediatric diabetes specialist nurse post implemented in 1995 was to avoid hospitalisation for children with newly diagnosed diabetes through the introduction of home management from diagnosis, when appropriate, and to minimise length of stay for those children requiring admission. To evaluate the effectiveness of this one aspect of a complex role, the authors undertook a quantitative study to examine the length of hospitalisation at diagnosis in the 2 years before (comparison group: $n = 40$ children) and 9 months following (experimental group: $n = 16$ children) implementation of the post (Lowes and Davis, 1997). The results showed a significant reduction of 3.5 days hospitalisation for newly diagnosed children who received input from the paediatric diabetes specialist nurse, five out of 16 children being managed completely at home. When looking at the extraneous variables that may have contributed to this outcome, there was no significant difference between the two groups in gender, age, family structure or clinical condition at diagnosis when defined by the blood pH or the requirement of intravenous therapy.

The study supported earlier findings (Swift *et al.*, 1993) that younger children are more likely to present in diabetic ketoacidosis. Eleven out of the 12 children under the age of 4 were ketoacidotic at diagnosis. All 12 children were initially hospitalised, but the length of stay for the children in the experimental group was significantly reduced, from 7 to 4 days.

When examining the adolescent population (11–18 years) across both study groups, 14 out of 21 adolescents were ketoacidotic at diagnosis. This may be due in part to teenagers being reticent about publicly questioning bodily functions and parents no longer being able to closely observe the behaviour of their teenager. Nineteen adolescents were initially hospitalised, but the length of stay for the experimental group was again significantly reduced, from 5 to 1 days.

When exploring the correlation between blood pH at diagnosis and length of stay across the total study population, children from two-parent families had a reduced length of stay when more clinically well at presentation. However, this variable was not found to influence the length of hospitalisation for children from single-parent families, which could suggest that single-parent families may require more intensive support if managed at home or have a greater need for an initial period of hospitalisation.

The findings from this study are supported by subsequent reports (Cowan *et al.*, 1997; Lowes, 1997) and suggest that paediatric diabetes specialist nurses can make a substantial contribution to improving the care of newly diagnosed children, if the nursing role enables these children to avoid or minimise hospitalisation, as recommended by the RCN (1994) and the Department of Health (1991). However, this is only achievable with the support and enthusiasm of an integrated multidisciplinary team, with shared beliefs about paediatric diabetes care and the benefits of home management for children with newly diagnosed diabetes.

References

Anderson, B.J., Auslander, W.F., Achtenberg, J. and Miller, J.P. (1983) Impact of age and parent–child and spouse responsibility sharing in diabetes management on metabolic control. *Diabetes*, **32** (supplement): 17A.

Baum, J.D. (1990) Children with diabetes. *British Medical Journal*, **301**: 502–3.

British Paediatric Association Working Party Report (1990) The organisation of services for children with diabetes in the United Kingdom. *Diabetic Medicine,* **7**: 457–64.

Cowan, F.J., Warner, J.T., Lowes, L., Ribeiro, J.P. and Gregory, J.W. (1997) Auditing paediatric diabetes care and the impact of a paediatric-trained diabetes specialist nurse. *Archives of Disease in Childhood,* **77**: 109–14.

Department of Health (1991) *Welfare of Children and Young People in Hospital.* (London: HMSO).

Department of Health (1994) *The Allitt Inquiry.* (London: HMSO).

Forsander, G. (1995) Family attitudes to different management regimens in diabetes mellitus. *Practical Diabetes,* **12**(2): 80–5.

Hamman, R.F., Cook, M., Keefer, S. *et al.* (1985) Medical care patterns at the onset of insulin-dependent diabetes mellitus: association with severity and subsequent complications. *Diabetes Care,* **8** (supplement 1): 94–100.

Koizumi, S. (1992) Japanese mothers' responses to the diagnosis of childhood diabetes. *Journal of Pediatric Nursing,* **17**: 154–60.

Lessing, D.N., Swift, O.G.F., Metcalfe, M.A. and Baum, J.D. (1992) Newly diagnosed diabetes: a study of parental satisfaction. *Archives of Disease in Childhood,* **67**: 1011–13.

Lipman, T.H. (1987) Length of hospitalisation of children with diabetes: effect of a clinical nurse specialist. *Diabetes Educator,* **14**(1): 41–3.

Lowes, L. (1997) Evaluation of a paediatric diabetes specialist nurse post. *British Journal of Nursing,* **6**(11): 625–33.

Lowes, L. and Davis, R. (1997) Minimising hospitalization: children with newly diagnosed diabetes. *British Journal of Nursing,* **6**(1): 28–33.

McClowry, S.G. and McLeod, S.M. (1990) The psychological responses of school-age children to hospitalisation. *Children's Health Care,* **19**(3): 155–60.

McEvilly, A. (1991) Home management on diagnosis. *Paediatric Nursing,* June: 16–18.

McEvilly, A. (1995) Liaison nursing – the diabetic home care team, in Kelnar, C.J.H. (ed.) *Childhood and Adolescent Diabetes.* (London: Chapman & Hall).

Metcalfe, M.A. and Baum, J.D. (1991) Incidence of insulin dependent diabetes in children aged under 15 years in the British Isles during 1988. *British Medical Journal,* **302**: 443–47.

Moyer, A. (1989) Caring for a child with diabetes: the effect of a specialist nurse on parents' needs and concerns. *Journal of Advanced Nursing,* **14**: 536–45.

Moyer, A.A. (1993) The specialist nursing care of children with diabetes. Unpublished PhD thesis, King's College, London.

Muller, D.J., Harris, P.J., Wattley, L. and Taylor, J.D. (1994) *Nursing Children: Psychology, Research and Practice,* 2nd edn. (London: Chapman & Hall).

Paediatric Diabetes Team, Newcastle and Gateshead (1993) *Diabetes. A Book for Children and their Families.* (Sussex: Boehringer Mannheim UK).

Pinkney, J.H., Bingley, P.J., Sawtell, P.A., Dunger, D.B. and Gale, A.M. (1994) Presentation and progress of childhood diabetes mellitus: a prospective population-based study. *Diabetologia,* **37**: 70–4.

Royal College of Nursing (1994) *The Care of Sick Children. A Review of the Guidelines in the Wake of the Allitt Inquiry.* (London: RCN).

Royal College of Nursing Paediatric Diabetes Special Interest Group (1993) *The Role and Qualifications of the Nurse Specialising in Paediatric Diabetes – a Working Party Report.* (London: RCN).

Royal College of Paediatrics and Child Health and the Joint British Advisory Committee on Children's Nursing (1996) *Developing Roles of Nurses in Clinical Child Health.* Report of a Joint Working Party. (Royal College of Paediatrics and Child Health: London).

Schneider, A.J. (1983) Starting insulin therapy in children with newly diagnosed diabetes. An outpatient approach. *American Journal of Diseases of Children,* **137**: 782–6.

Simell, T., Simell, O. and Sintonen, H. (1993) The first two years of type 1 diabetes in children: length of stay affects costs but not effectiveness of care. *Diabetic Medicine,* **10**: 855–62.

Swift, P.G.F., Hearnshaw, J.R., Botha, J.L., Wright, G., Raymond, N.T. and Jamieson, K.F. (1993) A decade of diabetes: keeping children out of hospital. *British Medical Journal,* **307**: 96–8.

Visintainer, M.A. and Wolfer, J.A. (1975) Psychological preparation for surgical patients: the effect on children's and parent's stress responses and adjustment. *Pediatrics,* **56**: 187–202.

Wearmouth, E.M. (1994) Family awareness and the diagnosis of diabetes. *Practical Diabetes,* **11**(3): 112–14.

17

HUB AND SPOKE MODEL OF AMBULATORY CARE

Sharon Stower

Health care services for children are constantly changing. Klein (1989) states that 'the NHS is like an Island of Stability in a sea of turbulent change' and it is within the context of such change that the health care services must be sustained, improved and remain appropriate to the changing needs of children and their families throughout.

Health care for children should be provided following the principle that, 'A service should be delivered to the child and not the child to the service.' In many ways, ambulatory care is an excellent way to ensure that the former is delivered. As mentioned below, the focus of ambulatory care can be delivered on a walk-in-and-out, one-stop basis during a day-time period. The setting for such ambulatory care can be delivered by different models set in both primary and secondary health care settings. For example, the polyclinic concept is one in which care such as medical health, dental health, physiotherapy, complementary therapy, chiropody and so on is all delivered to patients in their local community hospital or health centre. Another model is within a hospital environment, often in or attached to an outpatients clinic or centre, where similar services can be provided, as well as radiology and pathology services for example. Day surgical care can often also be attached to the centre. The focus with this model should be patient centred, by providing all the facilities in close proximity to where the patient's care is being carried out. The hub and spoke model is different again as care can be accessed on different sites and can be delivered by one or more 'providers', but by a collaborative approach. There is no preferred way except the way that best suits the client and/or local population. Each of the models has clear advantages and disadvantages; for example, many health centres/polyclinics cannot provide radiology and pathology services, although this is a developing trend. However, the advantage of geographical location to the patient often overrides any other deficits in this model of care. Patient-centred clinics in hospitals can often provide a variety of services, but they are usually located at different ends of the hospital, and co-ordinating appointment times is impossible. These services may provide long waiting times and patients may have to travel distances. With the hub and spoke model, a compromise situation can be reached by using the services of the larger (hub) unit and providing services locally. This model will now be explored in more detail.

Hub and spoke model of ambulatory care

The hub and spoke model of ambulatory care focuses on providing a safe qualitative service that is cost-effective, criteria that are becoming increasingly important. This model enables health care services to be much more primary care led, thus bridging the gap between primary and secondary care.

What is hub and spoke ambulatory care? There are different models that are common variations of a theme, but, simply defined, the 'hub' is the central point at which most activity is generated and the 'spoke' is the arm or bar joining up to the hub. So, in terms of hospital/health care services for children, the hub would be a large tertiary centre or district general hospital and the spoke a smaller unit that provides services for children and has a close working alliance with the centre or hub.

Ambulatory care embraces primary and secondary care and may comprise a number of different service components, which alter depending on the model and the client group concerned. The fundamental concepts of ambulatory care for children are well supported in the documents *Child Health in the Community* (NHSE, 1996) and *Flexible Options for Paediatric Care* (British Paediatric Association, 1993).

The children's services in Nottingham (Queens Medical Centre) and Grantham children's unit are a good example of a 24-hour hub and spoke service working collaboratively. This model can work particularly well in specific geographical areas, especially where the spoke unit is in a rural community.

The philosophy of the hub and spoke concept is to ensure that the services are child focused and that children and their families gain the benefits from the synergy of such units working together.

Resources can be shared, communication enhanced, and training and education of children's nurses and doctors improved through attachment to the centre and rotation, and there are many other clear benefits for children and their families.

These services should be provided locally, be accessible and have good parking/transport facilities, paying particular emphasis to the needs of children who are physically challenged or with special needs. This chapter discusses a specific approach to care for children that can work well in an ambulatory care setting using the hub and spoke model.

The present position

Across the country, children's services are being downsized under pressure to become more economically viable (Edwards, 1996; Payne and Martin, 1996). The major problem associated with this is that it reduces the spectrum of services for children and their families based in their own local communities. In this respect, the hub and spoke model is a qualitative and effective way of keeping services more locally based for families.

Smaller units often have problems in relation to sustaining their services, for example cost containment or retaining all the expert clinical skills of the doctors and nurses working in the smaller units. Factors such as audit, teaching and management can be problematic, research is limited, there is little or no real opportunity to specialise and some important services, for example skilled paediatric surgeons, anaesthetists and paediatric intensive care support, are often not available.

The 'hub' or large centre is important here for the viability of the 'spoke' unit because the activity from the centre (hub) provides most of the services that can be extended into other spoke centres. Thus economies of scale allow this model to be most cost-effective.

Services including a children's (and young persons') clinic, Outreach clinics in general practitioner surgeries or medical centres, unbooked walk-in clinics, medical assessment either through A&E or unbooked walk-in clinics, day surgery, ward attenders, community paediatric nursing care, mobile respite care, pharmacy, physiotherapy, occupational therapy and diagnostics are all aspects of care that can be provided locally for children with the management and co-ordination of such services being arranged from a hub unit (see Figure 17.1).

What does this mean for the children?

The focus on ambulatory care is that the care can be delivered on a walk-in-and-out, one-stop basis during a day-time period. This provides scope for a multiplicity of services to be provided, some of which will now be discussed in detail.

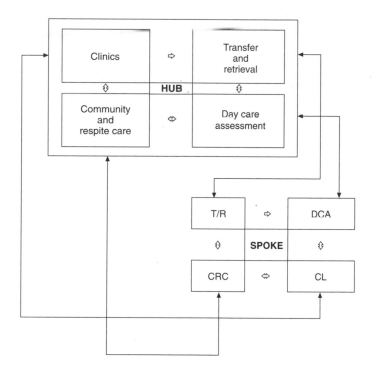

Figure 17.1 The relationships of the hub and spoke model of ambulatory care

Children's clinic

The children's clinic is the central focus of the majority of care for children and provides the link in the continuum of care between hospital, clinic and home (Stower, 1991).

Children's clinics are changing to accommodate a family-centred philosophy and are encapsulating as many professional services as possible at one attendance at clinic. For example, based in the children's clinic are the social worker, dietitian and community nurses for asthma, cystic fibrosis, diabetes and family therapy. Having these individuals working alongside medical staff means that treatments and advice can be given, as well as diagnostic tests carried out, all at one visit rather than requiring the family to attend on numerous occasions to see different professionals. Special attention should focus on young people. It is important that they have a separate area designated for them away from younger children, where they can read magazines or watch a video.

Nurse-led clinics and the development of the nurse practitioner role allow children to see their named nurse, for example, the asthma or respiratory care nurse, who can work independently but alongside the medical staff, giving invaluable advice to children and their families on inhaler techniques and so on. This developing role for children's nurses is important as it allows them to utilise their specialist skills and give high-quality service, time and care to the children.

With the ambulatory model of care, the question is what care/treatment and advice can safely and qualitatively be given to children in the day care ambulatory setting. This sets the scene for the potential role of children's nursing and the spectrum of care procedures that can be undertaken in the children's clinic.

An expansion to the clinic concept is the Outreach clinic, which takes care away from the hospital ambulatory setting into local general practitioner surgeries and medical centres. This is an excellent way of providing services even more locally in surroundings that are most familiar to the families. Again, the link here with the hospital ambulatory setting is that, with the Outreach model, the consultant from the hub extends out still further to provide this service. The children's nurse is also in attendance with other health care professionals to support as appropriate.

Family information centre

The provision of a family information service in the ambulatory setting plays an important role in keeping families informed and supported, especially when given news about their child's diagnosis. The ambulatory setting lends itself well to this: there should be easy access and information available on request. Such centres are described more fully in Chapter 4.

Unbooked walk-in clinics

Expanding the ambulatory model of care in the spoke unit, the unbooked walk-in clinic has many obvious advantages. As the title describes, this is a clinic (within the children's clinic) that is staffed by both medical and nursing staff for a given period on either set days or, usually, every weekday. The aim of this clinic is to give children access to the clinic without needing to wait on a waiting list to see a consultant. Three categories of child would use this service. The first group comprises children referred by their general practitioner for an 'urgent' or 'soon' opinion as the general practitioner is a little unhappy with the child's condition. The second group are those children with longstanding chronic problems who may have an acute exacerbation. The third group is made up of those children with minor trauma or requiring minor surgical procedures. The unbooked walk-in clinic often runs alongside another clinic or over a lunchtime period where direct access to medical staff can be guaranteed. This approach to care can reduce the need for the child's admission to hospital as an inpatient.

Telemedicine

The emergence of health telematics providing on-line consultation between the remoter location (spoke unit) and larger tertiary centre, in the form of video link-ups and telemedicine links, is also of benefit in aiding diagnosis. Tremblay (1996) identifies that the concept of telemedicine link-ups should be seen as the logical extension of possibilities that more remote links provide to professional staff, for example a consultant at the centre conversing with both a patient and nurse practitioner at the smaller unit by a video link-up. Such services could be to provide advice within the clinic setting or for the management of trauma in the A&E department. Where telemedicine is not afforded, the concept of telephone advice lines direct to the hub, manned by trained competent staff working to protocols, can be further explored.

These approaches suggest that people can more often be treated locally and, where possible, only using the specialist tertiary centre for specialist advice when necessary.

Telecare and information-based technology will, in its own way, change and develop different focuses on the delivery of health care. The health care industry itself will inevitably undergo substantial changes, and this may ultimately change the balance of power between patients and their care givers in the future.

Clinical protocols/pathways

Clinical pathways or protocols, which are clinically effective and research based, can provide an excellent framework for clinical practice, are cost-effective as they reduce unnecessary diagnostic tasks or interventions, and provide a safety net for staff working in the ambulatory care setting. This concept is of particular value to medical staff, especially when visiting the hub unit. For nursing staff, they provide a framework to assist in expansions to nursing roles when working within *The Scope of Professional Practice* (UKCC, 1992).

Organisation and multi-agency audit

The effectiveness of care needs to be proven. Evidence-based practice should ensure appropriate, effective and qualitative care for the client. This process needs to be evaluated to assess the level of effectiveness, and audit processes or audit trails are one way in which this can be achieved. The audit cycle does not have to be complicated or boring; it can be, and is, interesting, simple and extremely beneficial in identifying the effectiveness of outcomes of care.

Clinical protocols identify a critical pathway through which a child presenting with a specific illness or condition passes. For each stage or presenting feature, an outlined course of action is identified. This process ensures consistency, efficiency and quality in the outcome if it is proven by research or is an established route that has been clinically proven, and it should be the most cost-effective way of getting the child from point A to point B of the illness/condition.

Audit programmes can be set up to measure and monitor each step of this pathway. The audit programme will be to establish compliance with the desired route or measure the deviation and/or reason to deviate from the desired route. The audit process can also measure outcomes, that is, the differences between the desired outcome and the actual/perceived outcome of the child/parent. In this process, it is most common to measure all elements of care, which might include medical, nursing care, pharmaceutical therapy and so on (Figure 17.2).

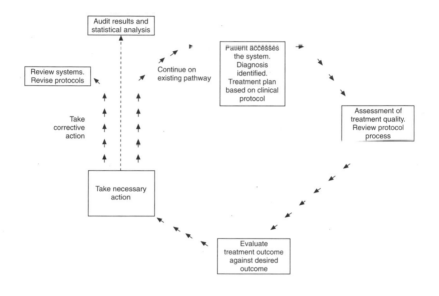

Figure 17.2 The audit cycle

The audit process/trail can exist in all areas where children visit or are cared for. This includes the A&E department, the children's clinic, the medical assessment/observation area and the community setting. As well as organisational audit, other key elements can be evaluated, for example by nursing documentation audit, record-keeping or environmental audit. Another area of record-keeping that is beneficial is in the monitoring of the number of children who attend the ambulatory setting direct from their general practitioner; this helps to assess the usefulness of the service and allows the development of informed changes to the service. The number of children attending A&E and being referred to the medical assessment/observation unit may be assessed; here for example, an analysis can be made comparing this model to the 'admission into hospital bed' model and the effectiveness of the children's community nursing team in respect of outcomes of clinical care.

The audit process requires multidisciplinary co-operation, but the benefits are that the services can then be modified around the specific requirement of children and their families. Patient satisfaction surveys are another useful tool to audit the quality of services.

Day care medical assessment/observation unit

In close proximity to the children's clinic is the day care assessment/observation unit. It is not essential to have the area next to clinic, but there are obvious advantages for doing so in that collaborative working between medical and nursing staff can take place. The area would function as a Monday–Friday day care ward. Surgical day surgery could take place here, providing that appropriately skilled surgeons and anaesthetists were available working alongside children's nurses. Another focus of the day care area would be for children requiring medical assessment. A child could be admitted from the children's clinic or the unbooked walk-in clinic and have the necessary investigations and examinations undertaken and a course of treatment identified.

The day care area can deal with a whole spectrum of paediatric interventions that do not require overnight attention; the child can always return the next morning for review or additional care treatment if necessary. If this is not appropriate, either admission to the hub for more serious concerns or follow-up with the specialist community nursing team can be arranged.

Ward attenders for blood tests or other diagnostic investigations would either attend the day care medical assessment area or children's clinic for their care. It is important that those children waiting for treatment or investigations in these environments should be encouraged to play: this may help in developmental assessments as well as relieve boredom.

Community children's nursing team and mobile respite care

The children and young people's charter recommends that all children have access to a team of community children's nurses (Department of Health, 1996). Unfortunately, many parts of the country do not have access to such a team. The ambulatory model of care, as is described here, relies on the availability and continuity of the children's community nursing team to provide ongoing care and support to families as well as linking in with the centre. In Nottingham, children's community nurses are both child-trained and possess a community-based qualification. Specialist nurses within this team are available to act as nursing consultants to other nursing and medical colleagues.

The community children's nursing team can provide care for children with some acute illnesses and chronic illnesses. It has proved to be an extremely high-quality and irreplaceable service for children and their families. One key focus of this service is the links between primary and secondary (or tertiary) care, which enhances a seamless service.

Working in tandem with the children's community nurse is the mobile respite care service. This is a small team of nurses providing care to children and their families, usually with long-standing chronically ill or physically challenged children. Care might be arranged to allow parents a rest or to go out shopping, perhaps undertaking nasopharyngeal suction or tube feeding in their absence. Both of these services support the ambulatory model of care.

The ill and seriously ill child

In any unit, the possibility of a seriously ill child attending either A&E or the day care unit must be anticipated. In the ambulatory care setting where no inpatient service is provided, appropriate services must exist to cover this potential occurrence. Facilities for immediate treatment at the spoke unit (depending on size and activity) might be appropriate, along with a facility for 'stabilising and holding', during which time the hub's retrieval or transfer team can be activated to take the child to the centre for ongoing care.

Staff development issues

The children's nurses working in the spoke unit can be employed by either the hub or a smaller spoke unit. However, attachment or affiliation to the hub means that the nurses have the ability to rotate through both centres. This is an important factor in the recruitment and retention of valuable, experienced children's nurses. Training and continuing education can also be enhanced with such an affiliation, as well as there being a strong leadership and management strategy for the organisation and development of all groups of professional staff.

For some, professional isolation can bring difficulties. For example, in the polyclinic setting in the community, staff can be isolated from their peers in hospital, which may affect their motivation and the ability to update their education. This having been said, there are opportunities for links between health clinics / centres and hospital education centres. Development opportunities exist but often need to be rigorously pursued. The hub and spoke model is one where this idea works well. Staff can be developed along with their colleagues in the hub, where networking and education can take place. This updating can then be returned to the system by the nurse rotating through the spoke unit; in a sense this is an iterative process that should always be ongoing.

The benefits of the hub and spoke model

The overall aim of any dynamic change in service provision must always centre around improving services to children and their families. If there is an economical imperative, this should be of secondary importance. Some would argue that the closure or reconfiguration of smaller units is not in line with this thinking, but when this occurs, for whatever reason, the hub and spoke model gives new life and vitality to the service. It is clearly a dynamic approach to the future vision of care delivery for children. The advantage of the hub and spoke model is that it can bring about effective improvements in the quality of care delivered locally, but through a larger centre where resources and economies of scale are concentrated. By affiliation with the hub, it provides an opportunity for children to have access to a very wide spectrum of services to meet their specific needs; this in turn enhances the smaller (spoke) unit's credibility as a local health care provider and, importantly, allows it to retain local pride.

Staffing issues

There can be some staffing difficulties at the spoke unit, but there is the ability to draw upon the larger mass of staff at the centre or hub unit. This is not always possible for short-notice staffing issues, for example sickness. However, the provision of a nurse-on-call system to support the spoke unit through this difficulty (particularly in the winter) can be most beneficial.

Another staffing issue relates to periods of low occupancy, which can and does occur; clearly, at least two Registered Sick Children's Nurses and Registered Nurses (Child) need to be available within the spoke unit at these times. It is often the focus by purchasing authorities on low occupancy of inpatient services that activates the considerations of moving from inpatient to ambulatory care services, and this is happening more and more across the country.

Disadvantages of the model

Disadvantages include the disenchantment of the local population, who see such a change as reducing local services. While centralisation is seen as improving the quality of care for families, by ensuring appropriate skills of staff and equipment at the large centre, it is perceived by the smaller unit as creating impotence, lack of local provision and reduction of the quality of service.

Health of the Nation targets

This model of care can facilitate health care professionals playing a vital role in the Health of the Nation targets. The importance of providing families with information relevant to both the child's diagnosis and general health cannot be overestimated. Ambulatory care can provide an ideal location for teenage clinics and other innovative ways of meeting these targets by locally based health gain programmes.

The charter for children and young people

As already mentioned, the charter standards play an important role in expanding and exploring services for children. Not all the charter standards are readily achievable, but many services are working towards the targets.

Conclusion

Hub and spoke models are different and dynamic. They challenge conservative ideas and preconceived views about how care should be delivered; they are workable and effective in delivering quality care to children and their families.

The impact of change in the smaller unit is often difficult for both staff and local communities to come to terms with. The political impact of changing services can create anger and frustration, particularly when there are implications for other services such as A&E, obstetrics and so on.

Assessment of the culture of both of the units is important to establish a way forward, as the process of managing change and changing existing practices can be a challenging prospect. Fradd alludes to 'an environment which is prepared to take risks and which recognises potential cultural differences, has innovative leaders amidst its team who will all support the affiliation model'. She goes on to add that 'staff who demonstrate flexibility and a desire to remain clinically credible, supported by a good communications strategy for all levels of staff within the internal organisation and the local community in the external world' (Fradd, 1995, p. 41) will all add to the potential success of such a venture of the hub and spoke model of ambulatory care.

References

British Paediatric Association (1993) *Flexible Options for Paediatric Care*. Report of a working group of the BPA Health Services Committee. (London: BPA).

Department of Health (1996) *The Patient's Charter – Services for Children and Young People*. (London: HMSO).

Edwards, N. (1996) Temperature rises for paediatrics. *Health Service Journal*, Feb: 24–5.

Fradd, E. (1995) Managing specialist units: case studies of acute children's units. *Nursing Policy Studies*, **12**.

Klein, R. (1989) *The Politics of the NHS*. (Harlow: Longman).

National Health Services Executive (1996) *Child Health in the Community, A Guide to Good Practice*. (London: DoH).

Payne, L. and Martin, C. (1996) Child benefit. *Health Service Journal*, July, 26–7.

Stower, S. (1991) The continuum of care. *International Journal of Health Care and Quality Assurance*, **4**(6): 4–9.

Tremblay, M. (1996) Telemedicine and society. *British Journal of Health Care Management*, **2**(3): 162–4.

UKCC (1992) *The Scope of Professional Practice*. (London: UKCC).

18

AMBULATORY CARE: MENTAL HEALTH ISSUES AND THE CHILD HEALTH NURSE

Michael Cooper

The health needs of young people are currently at the forefront of the research and policy agenda. Such interest, it seems, is of relatively recent origin, the health needs of adolescents previously having been largely ignored (West and Sweeting, 1996). West and Sweeting indicate that, in a recent study, one in five young people in the age range of 12–20 reported a long-standing illness, disability or infirmity, and in about half of these, activities were restricted. This is particularly significant when the established link between chronic illness and potential mental health problems is noted (Eiser, 1990). Clearly, then, the nature of the client group means that the nurse would not only be likely to encounter emotional and mental health problems, but would also be seen as having a role in:

> Enhancing the mental health of children and for tackling the less complex problems that occur so frequently. (Department of Health and Department for Education, 1995, p. 22)

The handbook goes on to say that the likelihood of having to deal with much more complex mental health problems may occur because of parents' unwillingness to take advantage of specialist services. This may in part be why, in developed countries, most children with emotional and behaviour disorders (80–90 per cent) do not reach specialist mental health services (Cox, 1993). Furthermore, if it is accepted that there is a link between untreated childhood mental distress and problems in adult life (Robins and Rutter, 1990), the case is strengthened for the child health nurse, among others, to have a role in mental health work.

Recognising and working with mental health problems

The specialist professionals involved in mental health issues use the discussion and analysis of individual cases as an accepted method of learning and supervision. Such an approach can be applied effectively to the exploration of their work and is therefore used in this chapter. Such descriptive analysis allows for illumination, imaginative speculation and the integration of theory and research. These skills are central to effective assessment and the implementation of appropriate care wherever mental health issues are engaged, particularly ambulatory care situations.

The following case studies offer a range of problems that would be referred to a community adolescent mental health service. The cases chosen focus mainly on depression and self-harm. Following the Health of the Nation (Department of Health, 1992) initiative, there is an increasing emphasis on developing, in all health care workers, skills related to the recognition of depression and the prevention of self-harm. The studies are presented as progressively more serious cases, Angela being the least severe and Susan the most troubled case. The cases aim to illustrate the work of such a specialist team and its limitations. This service is located within health service provision and has a mixed team of professionals, including psychiatrists, mental health nurses, a psychologist, a social worker and occupational/art therapists.

The theoretical models and therapeutic interventions are chosen because it is felt that elements of these approaches can be used by non-specialist practitioners dealing with mental health issues. The work of Winnicott, particularly the concept of 'holding' (Phillips, 1988), attachment theory (Bowlby, 1988; Ainsworth, 1991), family systems theory and cognitive-behavioural approaches will be used to illuminate the studies.

CASE STUDY 1

Angela is a 17-year-old, who is described, and describes herself, as, depressed. She sees her main problem as being her inability to 'get on with people', that is, to communicate in a normal social way. She can get on with some people, if she knows them well, but has never been able to share her troubles with her close friends. She believes that nobody would understand her and that she is not really interesting or worthy of their attention. She links her current difficulties to her relationship with her mother, which was always bad. It would appear that her mother was indifferent, unable to show love or even interest in her. When she talks about this, she initially connects with a deep sadness and then with frustration, resentment and anger:

'Everybody else I know had a caring Mum. Why did they, and why didn't I?'

'If your Mum does not like you, you can't be much good.'

In social situations, she believes that people will be critical of her and reject her. This leads her to be intensely anxious and therefore unable to initiate or follow along conversations. This in turn convinces her that she will be seen as no good.

Angela grew up in a northern town and the family moved to Newtown when she was 10. When she thinks back, she feels that:

'I was all right then, everybody knew everybody.'

When asked about the early times, she could identify friends but found it hard to recall specific happy times. However, when she thought more about it all more, she said that Dad was away a lot, and became very tearful. When asked what she would have liked Dad to do, she said:

'Care for me.'

And when asked how he could have shown his care she said:

'Notice what I have done.'

She sees herself as gradually losing all her friends and is beginning to distrust elements of even her closest relationships. It is as if she is not worthy of the attentions of others. Angela has difficulty with compliments; some people do compliment her but it's as if it 'stays on the top' and does not go in, and the next compliment just glances off; criticism, however, gets straight through. She feels that she shouldn't be like this.

Case analysis and discussion

It may difficult at first to be sure whether Angela has a serious mental health problem. This issue highlights the constant dilemma of exactly which clients an adolescent mental health service should be dealing with and what constitutes a serious mental health problem. Many young people would identify with aspects of Angela's problems. A number of young people feel awkward in social situations, lack confidence and find praise difficult to accept and criticism quite hurtful. The word 'depressed' was used to describe her, but this is a word often used by lay people and may not be the same as clinical depression. So how should the seriousness of her problem be judged?

The adult DSM IV criteria for major depression can also be used with adolescents and suggest the following:

- Depressed mood or loss of interest and pleasure, for at least 2 weeks duration, with no evidence of an underlying cause such as schizophrenia or hypothyroidism

plus at least four of the following:

- Feeling of worthlessness or guilt
- Impaired concentration
- Loss of energy and fatigue
- Thoughts of suicide
- Increased or decreased appetite with changes in weight
- Under- or oversleeping
- Retardation or agitation.

Angela certainly had an enduring depressed mood, feelings of worthlessness, agitation, loss of energy and fatigue, so even if it had not qualified as a clinical depression, it could be described as a depressive syndrome warranting mental health invention. The criteria suggested for childhood psychiatric disorder lack a degree of precision, and a lot is left to clinical judgement in terms of diagnosis (Pearce, 1996). It is considered that a child psychiatric disorder is present if there are anomalies in the child's behaviour persisting for at least 2 weeks and interfering with the child's everyday life. These anomalies are seen as a handicap to the child, to the carers or to both. The judgements need to be made mindful of the developmental stage and sociocultural context. Using these criteria, there is roughly a 10 per cent prevalence in the general population, which is much the same as for adults.

Given her history, it is likely that Angela would, at some time in childhood, have met the criteria for childhood psychiatric disorder. From her account, it is fair to speculate that her mother may well have had an undiagnosed depression. There is some concern that the children of depressed mothers are at risk of depression themselves and at greater risk of relapse when adults (Cox, 1993). In Angela's case, the transitions of adolescence have brought back to the surface elements of earlier distress and possibly the recurrence of an unrecognised childhood depression. There is some evidence, although not strong, to suggest that the rate of depressive disorder may be greater for this generation than previous ones (Graham, 1994).

Therapeutic strategies

In working therapeutically with Angela in an ambulatory care environment, the primary task would be to engage her in therapeutic alliance, that is, to build a working relationship that gives her the confidence to begin to look at her difficulties and how she might set about changing the more unhelpful views of herself and the world that she has developed. There are a number of ways in which Angela's problems can be construed. One perhaps well suited to her situation would be a cognitive-behavioural approach. Gilbert (1992) links the more conventional cognitive approach with an acceptance that our early experiences powerfully shape the way in which we see the world as we get older (Gilbert, 1992). Gilbert's model of cognitive structures comprises:

- automatic thoughts
- internal rules
- schema.

Automatic thinking is the most accessible and consists of the internal dialogue that individuals have. When people are depressed, this tends to be negative and self-defeating. There are clearly established patterns of negative thinking associated with depression. At a deeper level, it is thought that individuals have established rules for living their lives and interpreting events. The schema is nearer to the core idea of who we are, the central enduring beliefs about ourselves and others. Negative early life experiences increase the risk of a negative schema or self-view.

In a cognitive-behavioural approach, there would be a collaborative effort to help Angela to identify and challenge her negative automatic thoughts, internal rules and beliefs, and self-view. The aim would be to break the negative cycles of thoughts, feelings and behaviour, and to establish more helpful and adaptive patterns. Cognitive therapy starts from the premise that there is a clear link between how people think, how they feel and what they do. In people with psychological problems, these links often become negative cycles that lock the person into his or her depression or anxiety.

At the most immediate level, Angela's depressed mood and lack of confidence would be reinforced by constant negative automatic thoughts such as 'Everybody's looking at me; they think I'm stupid.' These would make her feel a failure, with the consequent emotions of frustration and sadness. This would in turn lead to the behaviour of avoiding social situations and put a strain on her relationship with her boyfriend. Her avoidance of social situations will increase her fear and dread of them because, without exposure to reality, the problems in her mind will just get bigger.

At a deeper level, there would be what are known as internal beliefs or rules, Angela's way of looking at the world. One of Angela's rules might be, 'If your parents don't like you, you cannot be worth much.' This might lead to other rules such as 'People will never like me just for who I am.' This view of the world may lead to behaviours such as always putting the wishes of others before her own and therefore making it more difficult to have her own emotional and psychological needs met. At a still deeper, more fundamental level would be Angela's central view of herself, or schema. Those who have had negative early experiences in their primary relationships tend to view themselves negatively as unable, unlovable, bad, selfish and ugly. This primary view of themselves gives shape to what they do, feel and think in life.

CASE STUDY 2

Stephen is 17 and lives at home with his mother, father and sister Jodie, aged 14. He has been referred to the community adolescent service by his general practitioner, who is concerned about his weight loss, self-harm and suicidal thoughts. At the initial assessment, Stephen presented as sad, anxious and dejected. He said that he was concerned that he needed to control himself and not to eat too much, although he needed some energy to think. He was worried that if he ate bad foods, he would in some way become tainted himself. He was very worried about his dog, who was now old and might soon die. In Stephen's view, the dog had a special role in the family, in that they would be united by having to focus on the dog, whose size made him very 'present' for all family members. His family concerned him as well; he was anxious that Mum and Dad might split up. He was also worried about his college work and said that he found it very difficult to concentrate. He was not sleeping well either and often in the night felt aware of an alien presence or force nearby, outside the house. Although the alien force did not seem to worry him, he was very concerned that he should be thinking these things.

He described his early life as uneventful at first, but that he could remember at about the age of 8 being very aware of thinking that 'there was little point to life; that things were born, lived a while and then died'. Although Stephen did not make the connection, it was about this time that his maternal grandfather died, and Stephen remembered very vividly seeing his grandfather in hospital very ill but still making a joke (while wearing the oxygen mask), pretending that he was a pilot. Another significant event for Stephen was the fact that the family had to move frequently because of his father's work. Although he had been unable to express it, the moves had made him angry and anxious. However, as a child he had felt powerless.

His relationship with his sister seemed healthy enough in that, deep down, they were fond of each other, although they were often in conflict. Father's work regularly meant that he was away, yet when he was at home, he would often spend a great deal of time on the computer. This worried Stephen, who saw this in part as evidence of conflict in his parents' relationship. Mother worried him as well: she seemed anxious and frail to him, as if she might have a breakdown, but paradoxically would be very tough on him and would drive him mad. Stephen was a deep thinker and found it difficult to mix with people who did not share his intensity. His appearance made him stand out, and he had a history of being bullied.

Case discussion and analysis

This is clearly a more obviously serious situation. The suicidal thoughts are indicative of high future risk, and there is also statistical evidence of young males, especially those who are unemployed, being at risk (Gunnell and Frankel, 1994). The seriousness of unrecognised depression and the potential for suicide are recognised in the Health of the Nation (Department of Health, 1992) initiatives on mental health, with the objective of reducing ill-health and death caused by mental illness. The initiative gives recognition to the importance of child and adolescent mental health and the serious implications for adult life of untreated mental health problems. Certainly, suicide rates among young people, especially young males, are causing significant concern. However, this is further complicated because this group currently makes the least contact with the health services (Gunnell and Frankel, 1994).

In the short term, it would be necessary for the therapist to engage quickly with Stephen in the hope of reducing this immediate suicide risk. In the longer term, it might be helpful for Stephen to view his problems within the context of his family, as many of his concerns centre on them. Family systems theory suggests that an individual's behaviour is best understood within the context of the social system, in this case the family (Johnson, 1995). It could be proposed that the main function of a family system is to survive, in much the same way as the main function of an individual body system is aimed at survival, through the use of homeostatic mechanisms. Stephen fears the threat to himself and the family in terms of his growing up and separating from them. In some systems theory approaches, the family system is divided into subsystems, which can then be analysed (Dykes, 1987). One of the critical elements in Stephen's situation, at the present time, is his relationship with his mother: the parent–child subsystem. Stephen and his mother have a very intense, anxiety-laden relationship. This family subsystem has unclear boundaries in that Stephen and his mother are enmeshed, or, less technically, too close. This shows itself in the fusion of Stephen's relationship with his mother, in that it operates predominantly from an emotional position rather than a mixed emotional and/or rational position (Johnson, 1995).

In terms of family systems, the parents' relationship is considered a subsystem – the spouse subsystem. In Stephen's family, the spouse relationship has elements of 'distancing', that is the couple manage the anxiety in their relationship by having less emotional and physical contact (Johnson, 1995). This natural phenomenon in relationships may be interpreted by Stephen as his parents growing apart, and this may be perceived as a precursor of family disintegration and, his most feared situation, his abandonment. In many ways, the sibling system is healthy in that Stephen and Jodie have the kind of relationship you might expect of a brother and sister of their ages. However, some of their natural conflicts and jockeying for position in the family may be made more stressful for Stephen because of his overall anxiety and fears.

Therapeutic strategies

Therapeutically, there are two clear tasks. First is to engage Stephen in a therapeutic relationship in order to minimise the risk of suicide, and second is, through that relationship, to support Stephen as he begins the process of separation from the family. The long-term therapeutic goal would be to provide Stephen with a 'secure base' from which he could rework the processes of separation and individuation on his way to adulthood. One of the criticisms of stage theories is that they suggest a tidy linear progression from one stage to another, but for everyone the process of individuation is a life-long process.

The important short-term therapeutic task in this crisis is to 'hold' Stephen in Winnicott's terms, to prevent his feared disintegration. Kaplan (1978) talks of Winnicott's 'holding' as:

> everything that happens to an infant which sustains him and produces wholeness and integration.

In a symbolic way, the therapeutic relationship would provide that 'holding' together. This holding, an essential task in adolescent work, became even more important in Stephen's case when, shortly after counselling started, the family dog died.

Although Stephen would not be aware of the dynamics of his behaviour, family systems theory analysis could be seen to offer a meaningful assessment of the situation, leading to appropriate interventions. The dog's death made Stephen more fearful that the family would fragment. It could be suggested that the family needs something to focus on, and Stephen's deterioration into the sick role gives them just that, thus holding them together.

After the dog's death, Stephen becomes quite depressed and withdrawn and is unable to do his college work. He feels as if he might 'lose his soul' and sees an 'apparition' of an old man through the condensation on his windows. His behaviour worries his parents, particularly his mother, and his general practitioner. Young people in crisis often fear they are going 'mad', and it is important for the skilled mental health worker to make some judgement about whether the 'unreal' experiences of the young person represent psychological crisis or the early stages of a more serious mental illness. The worker would use the resources of supervision and access to the child and adolescent psychiatrist to assist in making the judgement. In Stephen's case, the consensus view is that this is a young person in crisis, not one with a serious mental illness.

CASE STUDY 3

Susan, aged 16 years, was referred to the service by her social worker. The difficulties she presented included solvent abuse, problems with schooling and deliberate self-harm. It was considered that these activities were linked to a deeper psychological trauma, related to poor parenting experiences and sexual abuse. She had a long history of periods in care and fostering. On the whole, her experience had been of transient care situations, either with important adults who betrayed or abused her, or with those professionals who were 'paid to care'.

Her mother, Sandy, aged 32, had children from relationships with three different partners. Susan was the result of the second relationship, a short one that her mother ended, so Susan never knew her father. She thought of him often in a positive light and would have liked to make contact; her mother was against this. The third relationship had produced three other chidren. Susan had little contact with this family, which lived elsewhere. The stepfather was currently in prison as a consequence of his sexual abuse of Susan.

She had contact with the local drugs advisory service with regard to her solvent abuse and had a home tutor because she was not attending school. She had been seeing a psychiatrist but had stopped and would not see her again. When asked about how she saw things, she said that she did have problems and would like to stop solvents and cutting herself, and would like to be happy. However, she could not see this happening as she felt stuck in the same kind of groove and was unable to imagine what it would be like to be happy. When angry or frustrated, she would act out, becoming very impulsive, abusive and aggressive, and she had difficulty with most relationships. Her most meaningful relationship at that time was with a friend's mother: 'Wish she were my mum, like a mum should be.'

She observed that she felt sad and deadened and that the solvents stopped her thinking for a while. The cutting gave release to the tensions that built up but left scars. If other people saw these, they would think she was a loony, mad. Solvents were better because 'the scars are on the inside'.

Case analysis and discussion

Nabarro suggests that, of all the forms of childhood trauma, sexual abuse is probably the most damaging in terms of long-term psychological consequences. This study is included to demonstrate the factors that make such abuse so traumatic in some cases (Nabarro, 1992). Given the circumstances of Susan's early life, it is quite reasonable to postulate that Susan's mother was herself psychologically very needy and may have found it difficult to offer Susan the secure 'holding' experiences that would have helped her integrate. Her attachment to her mother is likely to have been anxious; the lack of a second care giver would have made things harder (Pearce,

1996). However, had her mother's longer-term relationship been a stable one and provided the family, including Susan, with a 'secure base', Susan's adjustment might have been made easier, although she would always have been vulnerable to psychiatric problems.

> Human beings of all ages are happiest and able to deploy their talents to best advantage when they are confident that, standing behind them, there are one or more trusted persons who will come to their aid should difficulties arise. The person trusted, also known as an attachment figure... can be considered as providing his (or her) companion with a secure base from which to operate. (Bowlby, 1979, p. 103)

However, instead of the secure base came a sexually abusive relationship from a violent and unstable parent figure. The betrayal by a trusted adult and the confusion it caused led to severe trauma, made worse by her mother's rejection of her when told about the abuse. In terms of trauma, these experiences left Susan in a very different place from the young people in the previous two case studies. The factors that protect or mediate against psychiatric disorder were clearly lacking. Such protective factors would include positive self-image, affectionate relationships, and supportive relationships with adults (Pearce, 1996). Other factors would include high levels of parental supervision, clear discipline, high IQ and a positive school environment with academic achievement and/or a special skill. Susan's life experience clearly lacked virtually all of these protective factors.

Therapeutic strategies

It was stated earlier that the most important therapeutic activity with young people who have the kinds of problem outlined in these studies is to engage them and build a therapeutic alliance. The success of such an activity depends on the skills of the therapist, the degree of psychological damage and the readiness of the young person to engage in the therapeutic process (Frank and Rush, 1994). In Susan's case, she found it very difficult to engage in one-to-one counselling. Given her history, this is understandable. Susan continued to use solvents and cut herself. Her impulsive behaviour and difficult history made her high risk in terms of suicide. Physical self-care and self-protection are acquired from early infancy

through the internalisation of parental attitudes during early physical care. Susan's history and the sexual and physical abuse left her
with a body experience that would make her prone to self-
destruction (Crowe, 1996; Orbach, 1996). The therapeutic task was
therefore one of containment. Bion developed the model of the idea
of a 'container' into which feelings are projected. In early relationships, the parent acts as the container: in therapy it is the role of the
therapist to contain the fears and emotions (Copley and Forryan,
1997). This containment reduces the risk of the client acting out his
or her fears and beliefs through self-harm. The containment of
Susan's behaviour would also reduce the anxiety in the other
professional workers and 'contain' them. This attempting to hold or
contain the anxiety around a case like Susan's is a central function
of a specialist mental health care worker. Given Susan's background, it is possible that she might not continue with individual
therapy; in the long term, she might only be contained within an
inpatient adolescent setting or by social services support.

Principles for mental health interventions by child health nurses

Some of the principles and processes used by specialist workers
could be adapted to assist the child health nurse.

The therapeutic relationship

The therapeutic relationship is central to the work of the specialist
mental health worker but is important in all nursing situations. The
quality of the nurse–patient relationship is dependent in part on the
nurse's awareness of her own attitudes and beliefs, and their effect
on nursing practice. The tendency to see self-harm negatively as
attention-seeking behaviour, and for the patient who self-harms to
evoke negative emotions in nurses, works against a positive relationship (Roberts, 1996; Sidley and Renton, 1996). The nursing relationship, even if transient, can be seen in terms of Bowlby's 'secure
base'. The nurse can be viewed as a trusted person who will come to
the patient's aid if needed. Illness and incapacity can produce
dependence and regressive behaviour. When this regressive behaviour produces passive dependence and compliance, it is labelled co-
operative. However, when the regressive behaviour is displayed as

anger, non-compliance and abusiveness, the patient may well be disapproved of and rejected by nursing staff. If the nurses' understanding of human behaviour (especially their own) allows them to be more understanding and tolerant, a therapeutic relationship is more likely to be formed, thus enhancing the patient's well-being. Such a nurse is likely to be able to contain and hold the patient's distressing emotions and thereby helping him. Even if it is necessary to set limits and boundaries on behaviour, these interventions are much more likely to be successful if they are motivated not by the nurse's distress and frustration but from a insightful understanding of the patient's needs.

Cognitive strategies

Although nurses would not normally be fully trained cognitive therapists, all nurses could use cognitive strategies in their therapeutic relationships with patients. In the case study above, Angela was asked how her father might show his care. This is a typical cognitive intervention. Rather than just assuming that they both know what a caring father was, the therapist asks specifically for Angela's unique view of what a caring father means to her. Her answer gives more clues about how Angela thinks about herself and the world (for example, 'He would notice me'). It may also give a clue about another 'internal rule' by which Angela judges the world: 'Caring people notice others.' This method of questioning is known as the Socratic method (Belsher and Wilkes, 1994). Socratic questioning seeks to enable patients to elaborate their assumptions and beliefs. Such elaboration may lead patients to recognise and then challenge their negative or unhelpful thoughts, assumptions and beliefs. The 'what?' question exemplifies this approach:

What is it about the situation that makes you uncomfortable?

Again, this style allows patients to elaborate their view of things rather than having the nurse make assumptions based on his or her own experience.

Recognition of depression and suicide risk

The recognition of depression could lead to a reduction in suicide attempts, as a substantial proportion of depressed children eventually attempt suicide (Kovacks, 1997). Another key area is the assessment of suicide risk. There are limitations to the research in this area, that is, to what we know empirically about suicide risk (Gunnel and Frankel, 1994; Williams, 1997). However, research can give general indicators for best practice. One of the common fallacies is that those 'who talk about it don't do it'. Research suggests that suicidal ideation is a good indicator of risk, as is a history of previous attempts. Asking direct questions to ascertain the degree of suicidal intent and the likelihood of a further attempt is a positive assessment strategy (Roberts, 1996). Certain psychological characteristics have been correlated with suicidal intent. These include hopelessness, impulsivity, hostility and aggression (Brent, 1997).

Although serious mental health problems should be treated by specialist services, there is increasing emphasis on improving the skills and understanding of all professional health care workers in the recognition and assessment of risk. Depression and self-harm are perhaps the most common mental health problems that the child health nurse will encounter. The ability to develop therapeutic relationships, recognise depression and assess the risk of self-harm would clearly be a positive and helpful extension of the role of the child health nurse.

References

Ainsworth, M. (1991) Attachments and other affectional bonds across the life cycle, in Parkes, C., Stevenson-Hinde, J. and Marris, P. (eds) *Attachment Across the Life Cycle*. (London: Tavistock Publications, pp. 33–51).

American Psychiatric Association (1996) *Diagnostic and Statistical Manual of Psychiatric Disorders*, 4th edn. Washington, DC: APA.

Belsher, G. and Wilkes, T.C.R. (1994) Ten key principles of adolescent cognitive therapy, in Wilkes, T.C.R., Belsher, G., Rush, J. and Frank, E. (eds) *Cognitive Therapy for Depressed Adolescents*. (London: Guilford Press, p. 35).

Bowlby, J. (1979) *The Making and Breaking of Affectional Bonds*. (London: Routledge).

Bowlby, J. (1988) *A Secure Base: Parent–Child Attachment and Healthy Human Development*. (New York: Basic Books).

Brent D. (1997) Practitioner review: the aftercare of adolescents with deliberate self-harm. *Journal of Child Psychology and Psychiatry*, **38**(3): 277–86.

Copley, B. and Forryan, B. (1997) *Therapeutic Work with Children and Young People*, 2nd edn. (London: Cassell).

Cox, A.D. (1993) Preventative aspects of child psychiatry. *Archives of Diseases in Childhood*, **68**: 691–701.

Crowe, M. (1996) Cutting up: signifying the unspeakable. *Australian and New Zealand Journal of Mental Health Nursing*, **5**: 103–11.

Department of Health (1992) *The Health of the Nation: A Strategy for England*. (London: HMSO).

Department of Health and Department for Education (1995) *A Handbook on Child and Adolescent Mental Health*. (Manchester: HMSO).

Dykes, C. (1987) The child the problem and the family, in Martin, P. (ed.) *Psychiatric Nursing. A Therapeutic Approach*. (London: Macmillan, Ch. 5).

Eiser, C. (1990) Psychological effects of chronic disease. *Journal of Child Psychology and Psychiatry*, **32**: 85–98.

Frank, E. and Rush, J. (1994) The therapeutic relationship with adolescents, in Wilkes, T.C.R., Belsher, G., Rush, J. and Frank, E. (eds) *Cognitive Therapy for Depressed Adolescents*. (London: Guilford Press, Ch. 5).

Gilbert, P. (1992) *Counselling for Depression Counselling in Practice*. (London: Sage, Ch. 3).

Graham, P. (1994) *Depression in Childhood and Adolescence*. Royal College of Psychiatrists Occasional Paper OP25. (London: Royal College of Psychiatrists).

Gunnell, D. and Frankel, S. (1994) Prevention of suicide: aspirations and evidence. *British Medical Journal*, **308**: 1227–33.

Johnson, B.S. (1995) *Child Adolescent and Family Psychiatric Nursing*. (Philadelphia: J.B. Lippincott, Ch. 5).

Kaplan, L.J. (1978) *Oneness and Separateness from Infant to Individual*. (New York: Touchstone/Simon & Schuster, p. 91).

Kovacks, M. (1997) Depressive disorders in childhood: an impressionistic landscape. *Journal of Child Psychology and Psychiatry*, **38**(3): 287–98.

Nabarro, E. (1992) The world turned upside down, responses to trauma in the family, in Noolan, E. and Spurling, L. (eds) *The Making of a Counsellor* (London: Routledge).

Orbach, I. (1996) The role of the body experience in self destruction. *Clinical Child Psychology and Psychiatry*, **1**(4): 607–19.

Pearce, J. (1996) Identifying psychiatric disorders in children, in Garralda, M.E. (ed.) *Managing Children with Psychiatric Problems*, revised edn. (London: BMJ Publishing Group, Ch. 1).

Phillips, A. (1988) *Winnicott*. (London: Fontana).

Robbins, L. and Rutter, M. (1990) *Straight and Devious Pathways from Childhood to Adulthood*. (Cambridge: Cambridge University Press).

Roberts, D. (1996) Suicide prevention by general nurses. *Nursing Standard*, **10**(17): 30–3.

Sidley, G. and Renton, J. (1996) General nurses attitudes to patients who self harm. *Nursing Standard*, **10**(30): 32–6.

West, P. and Sweeting, H. (1996) Nae job, nae future: young people and health in a context of unemployment. *Health and Social Care in the Community*, **4**(1): 50–62.

Williams, K. (1997) Preventing suicide in young people: what is known and what is needed. *Child Care Health and Development*, **23**(2): 173–85.

INDEX

Page numbers printed in **bold** type refer to figures; those in *italic* to tables